101

Things to Know If You Are Addicted to Painkillers

Michael McGee, M.D.

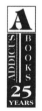

Addicus Books
Omaha, Nebraska

An Addicus Nonfiction Book

ISBN: 978-1-943886-94-4
Book design typography by Jack Kusler

This book is not intended to be a substitute for a physician, nor does the author intend to give advice contrary to that of an attending physician.

Library of Congress Cataloging-in-Publication Data
Names: McGee, Michael D., 1958– author.
Title: 101 things to know if you are addicted to painkillers / Michael D. McGee, M.D.
Other titles: One hundred one things to know if you are addicted to painkillers
Description: Omaha: Addicus Books, Inc., [2019] | Includes bibliographical references and index.
Identifiers: LCCN 2019015900 (print) | LCCN 2019016620 (e-book) | ISBN 9781950091140 (pdf) | ISBN 9781950091157 (kdl) | ISBN 9781950091140 (epub) | ISBN 9781943886944 (paperback)
Subjects: LCSH: Drug abuse. | Substance abuse. | Analgesics. | BISAC: MEDICAL / Pain Medicine. | SELF-HELP / Substance Abuse & Addictions / Drug Dependence.
Classification: LCC RC563 (ebook) | LCC RC563 .M34 2019 (print) | DDC 362.29—dc23
LC record available at https://lccn.loc.gov/2019015900

Addicus Books, Inc.
P.O. Box 45327
Omaha, Nebraska 68145
AddicusBooks.com
Printed in the United States of America
10 9 8 7 6 5 4 3 2 1

ii

To my sons, Shayan and Kian, who have taught me the most about love.

Contents

Foreword

Dr. Michael McGee brings so many facets of his knowledge and wisdom to the perplexing problem of addiction that the solutions seem quite clear—to not only addiction to painkillers, but to all addictive substances and destructive behaviors. Only someone like Dr. McGee with his training and own self-exploration could write this book. He brings together psychiatry, addiction medicine, pharmacology, meditation, spirituality, practical solutions, Internet resources, personal experiences, and patient narratives. All this in a clear, concise readable form.

McGee provides the reader with so many deep, yet simply stated principles and affirmations, that if practiced will lead to recovery from addiction as well as a rich, happy, and loving life. He uses his own formula for three phases of recovery— renunciation, healing, and self-realization. Throughout the book, he explains each phase and provides many concrete suggestions for step-by-step patient practice and achievement.

The excellent results of those who practice these principles have been validated by evidence-based research. I can almost guarantee that anyone who reads this book carefully and follows every step, preferably under the guidance of a capable mentor, will get sober and stay sober. And, of course they'll also let go of their addiction to painkillers as well as all else that brings pain to their lives.

Edward Kaufman, M.D.,
*American Academy
of Addiction Psychiatry*

Acknowledgments

Many thanks to my dear wife, Linda, who continues to provide unwavering love, support, and encouragement. You are my greatest blessing. I am so honored and humbled to be your husband.

Many thanks to Addicus Books publisher, Rod Colvin, my editor and newfound friend. Thank you for the idea for this book and the opportunity to write it. You have been incredibly supportive and encouraging. You have also helped me to be a better writer. I am deeply indebted to you. I am also grateful for the mysterious forces of fate that caused our paths to cross at just the right time.

I wish to acknowledge my many friends, my spiritual teachers, and my mentors. Your love, support, and guidance have helped me to realize the many blessings of my life.

Finally, I thank the millions of people who have walked the paths of recovery. I am so grateful for the generosity of so many who have given me the wisdom I've attempted to share in this book.

Although the world is full of suffering,
it is full also of overcoming it.

—*Helen Keller, 1880–1968*

Introduction

Congratulations! If you suffer from addiction to painkillers, you've come to the right place. You are reading the first words of a book that can help guide you to transforming your life from misery to joy! Don't despair, because there is hope. Millions of people have recovered from painkiller addiction to realize a life of joy. You can, too.

In fact, when you look back a year from now, you might even consider your addiction to have been a gift. Why? Because recovery will give you a life that is even better than the life you had before. It's hard to see this when you are in so much pain and your life is crumbling all around you. Have hope! With this book, the support of others, and daily effort on your part, you will not only recover, you will create an incredible life.

All you need is willingness to do the work of recovery. That is all. If you are willing, you will succeed. There is no one too "dumb," too impaired, or too hopeless to recover from addiction. Be willing to be humble and to open yourself up to being helped by others. You will need to be willing to be vulnerable, to connect with others who can help you, and to take the wisdom from those who have recovered from addiction. You will also need to be willing to follow the principles and practices outlined in this book. If you are willing, you will be on the road to recovery. If you are "done" with addiction to painkillers, let the lessons in this book guide you to the peace that comes with recovery.

Be patient. Recovery does not happen overnight. The thing that needs to change in recovery is everything. That includes your way of being in the world, how you see yourself and others, and how you behave. That is a lot! Accept that recovery takes time. Persist. Never give up. Greet setbacks as opportunities to learn and grow along the way.

You will find in this book a comprehensive approach to healing from addiction and living life addiction-free. Recovery is so much more than not using painkillers—it is about learning to live a fulfilling life of love. I pray that by faithfully following the 101 lessons in this book, you, too, will join the ranks of the addiction-free and realize a joyful life of recovery.

PART I
What You Need to Know about Addiction

1.   You can determine to what degree you might have an addiction to painkillers by asking yourself the questions below.

You may be wondering if you really do have an addiction. Here are some questions to ask yourself to make that determination. Be honest with yourself as you answer them. Let go of your fear of the truth. Remember that when it comes to addiction, seeing the actual truth of things is the first step to setting you free.

It is likely that you have an addiction to painkillers if you answer "yes" to two or more of these eleven questions:

1. *Do you take painkillers in larger amounts or for longer periods than prescribed?* Do you ever take painkillers other than exactly as prescribed?

2. *Do you want to reduce or stop using painkillers but just can't?* Do you try to set limits on their use, but end up using more than you planned, or more often than you intended?

3. *Do you spend a lot of time getting, using, or feeling bad from using painkillers?* Do you go to multiple doctors for prescriptions, try to get other people's medications, or buy painkillers off the street? Do you think about how bad you felt after your last use? Have you been dishonest with others about your painkiller use? Have you tried to hide or minimize your use?

4. *Do you have cravings to use painkillers?* Cravings are part of addiction. When you run out of pills, do you start craving them?

5. *Are you unable to manage responsibilities at work, home, or school because of painkiller use?* Have you lost jobs? Forgotten to complete tasks at work? Have you missed family functions or showed up impaired? If you're in school, have your grades dropped?

6. *Do you continue to use painkillers even when it causes problems in relationships with family or friends, with the law, or with your job?* Do you have trouble getting along with co-workers, teachers, friends, or family members? Do others complain about how you act, or comment on how you have changed? Do you have money problems due to loss of income or increased spending on painkillers?

7. *Have you given up important social, recreational, or work-related activities because of painkiller use?* Are you isolating socially because of time spent addicting or hiding your painkiller use from family and friends? Have you lost interest in family, friends or activities you used to enjoy?

8. *Do you use painkillers again and again, even when it puts you in danger?* This can include driving or operating heavy machinery while intoxicated. Do you purchase illegal drugs from a drug dealer?

9. *Do you continue to use, even though your painkillers cause physical or mental problems?* Do you have mood swings or bouts of anger and irritability? Are you fearful, anxious, or paranoid for no clear reason? Do you appear lethargic or "spaced out?" Does your energy level fluctuate from exhausted to energetic? Have you lost your motivation?

10. *Have you developed tolerance so that you need more painkillers to get the wanted effect?* After you take a narcotic for a period of time, your brain becomes used to the narcotic. You need more and more to get the same effect you got in the beginning.

11. *Have you developed withdrawal symptoms that are relieved when you take more of the painkillers?* When you stop taking painkillers, do you feel achy, anxious, depressed, nauseous, sweaty, chilled, or tired? Have you been feverish? Do you have cramps? Have you been irritable or nervous?

In addition, there are other signs of addiction to painkillers that you may have experienced. They include:

- Bloodshot eyes
- Dilated or constricted pupils
- Slurred speech
- Impaired coordination
- Bad breath
- Unusual odors on your body or clothing
- Shakes
- Weight loss or gain
- Poor grooming or hygiene
- Nodding off

Behaviors that go along with addiction include:

- Stealing money, possessions, or prescription drugs
- Behaving illegally
- Borrowing money
- Sleeping erratically
- Arguing with friends or relatives
- Behaving erratically
- Having accidents around the home, at work, or in the car
- Isolating from friends and family
- Hanging out with other victims of addiction
- Lying about one's activities or whereabouts
- Unexplained trips out of the house

Addiction erodes character. You may have noticed yourself becoming more self-centered, secretive, manipulative, or dishonest. You may have abandoned your moral compass. You feel like you aren't yourself anymore. If you see a negative change in your personality, it is likely due to addiction.

You've probably recognized these changes in yourself on some level, so looking honestly at the truth is probably a relief. By seeing your behavior clearly, you can now act to address your painkiller addiction. Don't despair! There is help and hope. That is exactly what this book is all about.

2. If you are addicted to painkillers, you are not alone.

You may be wondering, "How did I get myself into this mess? What is wrong with me?"

Know that you are not alone. Right now, millions of people just like you are suffering because of their addiction to painkillers, part of a class of drugs known as "opioids."

When you take into account all addictions, including food addiction, about 100 million people suffer from addiction. That's nearly one out of every three people in the United States. The fact is that addiction has reached epidemic proportions in our society. When you go out, look to your left and look to your right. The chances are you will be looking at someone else who has fallen into addiction.

Each year in the United States, approximately 72,000 people die from the consequences of opioid use disorder. When doctors prescribe painkillers, about one out of every ten patients will develop an addiction to painkillers. As you can see, addiction to painkillers is very common.

If you were prescribed painkillers, did your doctor tell you that you had a 10 percent chance of developing an addiction? Did he or she tell you that if you did develop an addiction that you would suffer terribly, and that you would face the risk of actually dying of your addiction? Likely not.

One of the reasons that we have an opioid epidemic is that some of the makers of painkillers heavily marketed these drugs to doctors without emphasizing the risks of addiction. People don't like to be in pain, and doctors want to help. So doctors prescribed painkillers liberally to people for many years without taking into account the risks of addiction. That is a big reason why you are not alone in your battle with addiction to painkillers.

Addiction is a highly treatable disease. Millions of people have gone through what you are going through and have come out the other side into recovery.

Also, if you have attempted treatment before and have relapsed, you are not alone. Addiction can be thought of as a chronic illness with relapses and remissions, just like diabetes or congestive heart failure. Between 40 to 60 percent of people receiving addiction treatment experience episodes of readdicting. Learning to be in recovery is like learning to walk as a toddler. Just as it takes several attempts for a young child to learn to walk, it takes some people a number of attempts to stay in remission from addiction. The good news is that with practice and persistence, combined with good treatment, you can join the ranks of millions of people who have overcome addiction.

3. Addiction is not a choice.

Although you may have chosen to use painkillers, you did not choose to develop an addiction. Addiction develops in genetically vulnerable people when their brains experience excessive reward, such as that with painkillers. You most likely have that genetic vulnerability.

Let's look at how that happens. Your brain has a drive-reward system that is essential for your survival. When you have experiences that promote survival, such as eating food or having sex, your brain secretes pleasure molecules called endorphins to reward you for your behavior. Your brain then drives you to repeat these pleasurable experiences in part through a drive molecule called dopamine.

Your addiction is due to a disturbance of your drive-reward system. You experience excessive desires and urges to repeat using painkillers. You experience these desires and urges as cravings and compulsions—feeling driven to take pills. Your brain is saying, "I want painkillers!"

Cravings and compulsions arise out of an imbalance of a number of brain transmitters, chemicals that transmit signals between nerve cells in the brain, including the transmitter do-pamine. It regulates attention, movement, learning, and emotional responses. It also enables you to move toward rewarding behavior. These chemicals take away your ability to act freely according to what is best for you in the long run. When you are in the middle of your addiction, you lose your ability to choose.

For most people, addiction arises out of attempts to numb pain. Think about yourself. Is this true for you? What was the pain that motivated you to try painkillers? Was it physical pain or emotional pain? If it was emotional pain, was it anger, anxiety, stress, grief, uneasiness, or maybe a vague desire for "something more?"

Whatever the case, when you used painkillers, they took away your pain and left you feeling good. Painkillers are very rewarding. When they wear off, your brain remembers how good they felt and drives you to want more.

As you continued your use of painkillers, you probably noticed two things: One, you likely noticed that you needed more painkillers to get the same effect. That is called tolerance. You probably also noticed after a while that you felt bad when the painkillers left your system. That is called withdrawal. Both tolerance and withdrawal result from changes in your brain. After a while, you probably switched from using painkillers to feel better to using them to stop from feeling worse. Rather than your brain saying, "I want to use painkillers," now your brain is saying, "I need to use painkillers" to prevent feeling worse. Switching from "want to" to "need to" is a sign of your brain suffering from withdrawal.

Tolerance and withdrawal are your brain's ways of trying to keep you in balance. In a sense, addiction is when two parts of the brain are working against each other. You can think of your brain as being in conflict with itself. One part of your brain, the brain's drive-reward system, says "I want painkillers!" It also wants to reward you with good feelings when you take painkillers. But another part of your brain is saying, "Let's stay neutral and even." The brain does not want to be in ecstasy all the time; it neutralizes the good feelings so that you can be ready to be rewarded by other important survival behaviors.

Although addiction is not a choice, recovery from addiction is. You can choose recovery today, right now! You have the capacity to choose to ask for help. You can empower yourself to get treatment for this potentially fatal illness. Later on in this book we will talk about all the things you can choose to do to rescue your brain from addiction.

Commonly Abused Opioids

Generic Name	Brand Name
• Codeine	Available only in generic form
• Fentanyl	*Actiq, Duragesie, Fentora, Abstral, Onsolis*
• Hydrocodone	*Hysingla, Zohydro ER*
• Hydrocodone/ acetaminophen,	*Lorcet, Lortab, Norco, Vicodin*
• Hydromorphone	*Dilaudid, Exalgo*
• Meperidine	*Demerol*
• Methadone	*Dolophine, Methadose*
• Morphine	*Kadian, MS Contin, Morphbond*
• Oxycodone	*OxyContin, Oxaydo*
• Oxycodene and acetaminophen	*Percocet, Roxicet*
• Oxycodone and naloxone	

---

4. Addiction may result from numbing emotional pain.

There is one thing we all share—we all want to feel good and to not feel bad. In fact, almost everything we do is aimed at trying to feel good. We all have three core ego needs (The "ego" refers to your sense of self—"I," "me," or "mine"—that is concerned with your survival.) The three ego needs are: to feel safe, to feel comfortable, and to feel connected to others. Beyond this, we have our higher need to love. When all these needs are met, we feel good. When one or more of these needs are not met, we feel bad. We call that bad feeling pain. No one wants to be in pain.

Emotional pain gets a bad rap. Although it brings discomfort, pain is not necessarily bad. In fact, pain has a purpose.

Pain sternly tells us something is wrong that we need to fix if we can. It grabs our attention. It motivates us to meet our needs for safety, comfort, connection, and love in order to restore our well-being.

Opioid Addiction Is Deadly

More than 2 million people in the United States have an opioid use disorder, which is caused by prolonged use of prescription opioids or illicit ones such as heroin and fentanyl. Opioid use disorder is a serious chronic illness—individuals who suffer from it have a twenty-fold greater risk of early death due to overdose, infectious disease, trauma, and suicide.

—*National Academies of Science, Engineering, and Medicine*

For many people, painful periods in their lives are often the greatest times of growth and transformation. This is why many spiritual teachers teach us to value painful times.

The bottom line is that pain is grossly underrated and underappreciated. Over and over again, pain saves our lives and teaches us how to live more skillfully, if only we will learn from our painful experiences. That is why some people say the secret to a long and happy life is skillful pain management. When we resolve pain skillfully in ways that restore our safety, comfort, connection, and our capacity to love, we restore our well-being. To love yourself is to act to enhance your well-being, to resolve pain skillfully is to resolve pain with love.

So where does addiction come into all of this? When you got hooked on painkillers, you first took them either to numb physical pain or to numb emotional pain. You took painkillers because they made you feel really good. You may have noticed that painkillers quelled feelings of anxiety, anger, emptiness, loneliness, or boredom. You were bathed in the warm, euphoric glow that painkillers give at the beginning.

The problem is that as time went by, the rewards of painkillers faded away. You probably found you had to take more and more as you tried to re-experience that first high. There is a solution. That solution is called "recovery." Recovery will teach you how to manage your pain without numbing it with addiction.

5. Addiction can also result from treating legitimate physical pain.
Treatment for physical pain is another factor that may contribute to addiction. You may be one of the millions of people whose addiction started when their doctors prescribed painkillers for legitimate physical pain. Opioids, or painkillers, are very effective for treating some forms of pain. People don't want to be in pain, and doctors want to help. Thirty years ago, several factors led doctors to overprescribe painkillers for physical pain, leading to the current opioid epidemic:

- Drug companies spent a lot of money trying to get doctors to prescribe painkillers.

- Doctors were not as aware as they are now of the addictive potential of painkillers.

- The field of pain management was not as evolved as it is today in terms of non-narcotic approaches to treating long-term pain.

- Many doctors often prescribed many more painkillers than people needed, leaving leftover painkillers in millions of medicine cabinets for others to take.

You may have been one of those people who noticed that painkillers not only helped your physical pain, but they also made you feel good, numbing painful emotions.

If you suffer from chronic pain, then your risk of addiction is even greater. The longer you take painkillers, the greater your risk of addiction. The severity of your pain may have also played a role in your addiction; you may have needed more painkillers to control your pain than someone with less pain.

We now know that there are better ways to manage physical pain and reduce the risk of painkiller addiction. First, doctors need to estimate the risk of addiction. If you have any other addictions or if you have a family history of addiction, then your doctor should know that you are at a higher risk of developing an addiction. Regardless of the degree of risk, doctors need to avoid prescribing narcotic painkillers if at all possible. They also need to prescribe the minimum amount necessary and transition patients to non-narcotic pain medication as quickly as possible. We also know now that we can treat chronic pain effectively without narcotics by providing combinations of other medications that reduce pain; also non-medication treatments can be added, including acupuncture, massage, physical therapy, and psychotherapy.

If you suffer from chronic physical pain, take heart. You can work with a pain management team to treat your pain using nonaddictive medications and other treatments. One key thing to know is that you don't have to suffer anymore. Your caregivers can work with you to minimize your physical distress and help you live with any remaining physical distress.

6.   Addiction is not your fault.

No one chooses to become addicted. You probably have genes that make you vulnerable to addiction. Your upbringing, environment, and stress also played a role in your becoming addicted to painkillers. Remind yourself that you didn't choose your genes, your parents, your upbringing, or where you grew up. Not only did you not choose your brain's makeup, you also did not choose much of its programming during childhood. So much of what happens to us is beyond our control. If you look closely, you will see that you don't even choose the thoughts or feelings that arise in your awareness from moment to moment.

In fact, all we really have control over to some degree is what we pay attention to, our attitude, and some of our more thoughtful, considered actions. Most of our actions are automatic, habitual, and reflexive, beyond our conscious choice.

It's not your fault that your brain really liked the way painkillers made you feel. It's not your fault that your brain naturally created a desire to repeat that experience. That's what brains do. They drive us to repeat rewarding experiences. The problem is that your brain developed an overly strong desire for painkillers, called a craving. Along with the craving came an overwhelming urge to take more painkillers. You did not choose to have these strong cravings and compulsions. These cravings and compulsions are symptoms of a disturbance in your brain's drive-reward system because of your genetic vulnerability to addiction. In the midst of your cravings and compulsions, you lost part of your free will. You lost your capacity to choose what is best for you even though you realized painkillers were causing more harm than good. It's also not your fault that you took painkillers to feel good and to numb pain. Everyone does things to change the way they feel. That is normal. Remember, we all want to feel good and to not feel bad. You're not the only one who took a substance in order to feel better. The next time you walk into a convenience store, look around you. On one wall there is alcohol. On another, there are caffeinated drinks. The aisles are full of crunchy carbs and sugary sweets. Behind the counter are the nicotine products. We might as well change the name of convenience stores to consciousness alteration stations. All these products affect the way we feel.

Millions of people just like you have also taken painkillers to relieve physical pain. About one out of ten people develop an addiction to painkillers. And just like you, they did not choose to become addicted. Although you did make that initial choice to take painkillers, I know for sure that you didn't say to yourself, "I want to devastate my life by becoming addicted to painkillers." You may have even known in the back of your head that there might be a risk of developing an addiction, but you probably thought it wouldn't happen to you. You just wanted to feel well.

You didn't choose to lose your capacity to choose. Something happened to your brain when it was exposed to painkillers. You've probably done a lot of things that you regret because of your addiction. Although you want and need to hold yourself accountable, don't beat yourself up. Realize that forces not of your choosing drove you to addict.

Although addiction took away your capacity to choose to not use painkillers, you still have a choice: you always have the choice to empower yourself by humbly asking for help. You have the capacity to choose recovery. You have the choice to see and acknowledge the truth of things. You have the choice to treat yourself and all your experiences with a compassionate attitude and to renounce shame. Realize that you have the choice to ask for help. Recognize that you have this choice, and choose recovery. We'll talk more about recovery later in Part IV.

7. Many factors contribute to addiction.

Addiction, like many other illnesses, is an illness with many contributing factors. Remember that addiction follows pain. Addiction arises out of attempts to use addictive substances or behaviors to relieve pain, even if it is just the pain of cravings and withdrawal symptoms. The more pain there is, the greater the vulnerability to addiction.

Pain comes in many forms. One form is stress. Stress is a huge factor in developing addiction. Consider the example of many Vietnam veterans who developed an addiction to heroin when they were in Vietnam. When they came back home, nine out of ten were able to stop using heroin once they were out of the stressful war zone environment. Unfortunately, about one out of ten Vietnam veterans continued to have an addiction to heroin when they came home. These veterans likely had a greater genetic vulnerability to addiction. Genetics play a big role in addiction. You may well have family members or relatives who also suffer from addiction. Addiction tends to run in families.

Another factor that contributes to addiction is "trauma." Trauma refers to deeply distressing events that are physically or emotionally harmful. Sexual, physical, and emotional abuse, and bullying are all traumas than can cause lasting harm. Trauma creates a lifetime of pain for many people. About 70 percent of people who suffer from addiction suffered from trauma, usually while growing up.

One form of trauma that is particularly damaging is neglect, either physical or emotional. If you were neglected growing up, then you probably suffered damage to your sense of yourself as a capable, whole, and lovable person. You also probably didn't receive the training you needed to learn how to safely and effectively love and be loved. You did not fully develop your capacity for healthy, loving relationships. People who were neglected as children often enter adulthood feeling broken and emotionally crippled. Their pain then lures them into numbing themselves with potentially addictive substances and behaviors. In fact, the more trauma you experienced growing up, the greater your risk is of developing addiction. The more trauma, the more pain, and the more damage to your capacity to cope and to heal.

Psychological disability also contributes to addiction. People with psychiatric illnesses other than addictions have higher rates of addiction. This may be due to increased psychological pain, impulsivity, or impaired coping skills. Other social forces also contribute to your vulnerability to addiction. Poverty is stressful, so it is not surprising that poor people are more vulnerable to addiction. Addiction is also more common in violent, high-crime neighborhoods.

You are also more vulnerable to addiction if your friends and family members use addictive substances. If this is the case, then using painkillers or other addictive substances may seem normal to you. Peer pressure may have made using painkillers irresistible, as you may have felt you needed to take them to fit in. Addiction for many is like a poisonous stew with several "ingredients."

8.   Addiction creates more pain in your life.

You have probably discovered that addiction, rather than resolving pain, increases pain. At first there was the pain that drove you to use painkillers, whether it was physical pain or emotional pain. But now you experience new pains in the form of cravings, withdrawal symptoms, and the painful consequences of addiction, such as financial losses and legal troubles. At this point, you may have used painkillers to relieve yourself of these pains as well. You got caught in a vicious cycle of numbing pain with something that created even more pain. That's what addiction does.

You know all too well about the pain of cravings. It hurts to really want something badly and not get it. People call this the "pain of desire." Buddhists talk about the pain of grasping for something you don't have. They spend years in meditation and the practice of restraint to get to the point where they can be at peace in the face of strong desires. As part of your recovery, you, too, will need to learn to work skillfully with your cravings.

You also know about the pain of withdrawal. Your brain has gotten used to having painkillers in your bloodstream. While withdrawal is not fatal, it is very uncomfortable, like a very bad case of the flu. Your cravings and withdrawal symptoms have likely trapped you in a corner where you feel you can't get out. Don't worry, you can get beyond these pains. With appropriate treatment, the pains of cravings and withdrawal go away with time.

Addiction itself is traumatic. Almost everyone suffers from painful consequences of their addiction. You have likely suffered from one or more painful losses. You are not alone in this. People lose jobs, relationships, and possessions. They suffer negative health consequences, such as HIV, hepatitis, and infections. They suffer injuries from accidents and overdoses. By engaging in illegal behaviors to support their addiction, they suffer from legal consequences. People also suffer from the loss of the joy that friends, hobbies, and recreational activities once provided. This is because their addiction narrows their lives down to the cycle of using painkillers, recovering from use, craving more painkillers, and seeking out more painkillers to use again. Addiction squeezes the joy out of life.

9. Addiction creates shame, which fuels addiction.
Shame is one of the most destructive human emotions. Where there is addiction, there is shame. One feeds the other. As your addiction progresses, there is more shame. And as your shame builds, there is more addiction.

You likely have experienced both guilt and shame as a result of your addiction. That is because addiction has caused you to behave destructively. You have likely hurt both yourself and others. When we hurt ourselves and others, we feel bad about what we have done. That is guilt.

We feel shame when we feel bad about who we are. If you feel shame, it is because you feel you are bad because of the bad things you have done. This only fuels addiction, because shame drives you to punish yourself by hurting yourself even more. What better way to hurt yourself than by continuing to addict? Addiction is very powerful, because it makes you feel better for the moment while also satisfying your unconscious desire to hurt yourself because of your shame.

To heal from your addiction, first you must shed your shame. How do you do this? It helps to talk about it—share your "darkest" secrets with someone you trust, such as a therapist. You will learn that you're not that different from thousands of other people. Also, stop taking negative messages from your brain personally. Realize that you do not choose the thoughts, feelings, and perceptions that your brain generates. You also don't choose the urges that you experience. Your brain is generating all of these things in your awareness beyond your conscious control. Just because your brain has been hijacked by drugs and causes you to do bad things does not mean that you are a bad person. Keep in mind, however, that to heal and to be whole, you must still take accountability for your behavior—even your addiction-driven behavior.

"Shame is the intensely painful feeling or experience of believing that we are flawed and therefore unworthy of love and belonging. Something we've experienced, done, or failed to do makes us feel unworthy of connection."

Brene Brown, Professor
University of Houston

Second, see who you really are—this is the pure field of Awareness in which experience arises. I use the word "Awareness" most reverently—that's why I capitalize the word. You'll note I do the same with other "sacred" terms throughout the book. As that pure Awareness, you are a miracle of immeasurable value. You are a sacred being, just like everyone else. The problem is not you. It is the diseased thoughts, feelings, and urges generated by your addiction.

Third, replace shame with compassion. Although you can't control the thoughts, feelings, and urges that your brain generates, you do have control over your attitude toward your brain. Substitute shame with compassion for yourself. Be like a loving parent is to their sick child. Have compassion for your sick brain. As you substitute shame with compassion, you empower yourself to take care of yourself.

Fourth, armed with self-compassion and mindfulness, take care of yourself. Get help to stop hurting yourself and others. This will reduce your shame. While you do not have complete free choice when in the grips of strong cravings and compulsions, you do have a choice now. You can choose recovery. You can choose to ask for help. You can choose to reach out and connect with others who can help you when

Narcan Can Save Your Life

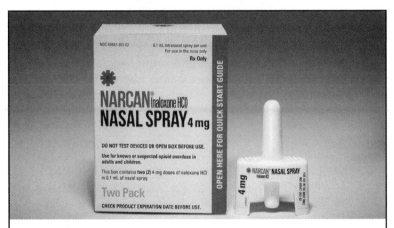

Narcan is emergency medication that can save the life of someone who overdoses on opioids, including heroin and fentanyl. It works in the brain to block the absorption of opioids. The medication comes as a nasal spray. It works in two to three minutes.

If you suspect someone has overdosed on opioids, spray Narcan into one nostril and call 911. If the person does not improve in two to three minutes, spray a second dose into the other nostril.

The Surgeon General of the United States recommends keeping Narcan on hand to give to those at elevated risk for an opioid overdose. Anyone who:

- misuses opioids
- has an opioid addiction
- has completed a treatment program and is not using methadone, buprenorphine, or naltrexone to prevent readdicting
- has recently been discharged from emergency care for an opioid overdose
- has recently been released from incarceration with a history of opioid abuse

Narcan is the brand name for naloxone. It is available without a prescription in virtually all pharmacies in the United States. The cost is covered by most insurance plans.

you are in the midst of your compulsions, cravings, negative thoughts, and destructive feelings. Commit to acting with love in everything that you say and do. Commit to asking for help so that you don't harm yourself anymore. The practices of awareness, compassion, and asking for help will resolve your shame. Be patient and persistent. You will need to practice these skills repeatedly and consistently for the rest of your life for them to be effective. If you do, you will keep shame at bay. If you do not, shame will creep back in like a cancer, bringing addiction with it.

10. Addiction will destroy your life if you continue to addict.
One thing you should be very clear about is that your painkiller addiction will destroy your life if you let it progress. In fact, about 50 percent of people with painkiller addictions end up dying of overdoses or other fatal consequences of their addiction. Your choice is to either choose recovery or lead a damaged life that will likely end before it should.

Your addiction is the only illness that will tell you that you are okay when you are not. This is called denial. Your brain needs the painkillers to feel normal, so it will lie to you. Or, it will give you reasons why you need to keep taking painkillers, such as telling you that your problem is not that bad, that others are overreacting, or that you have no other option. Addiction is deceitful.

Don't let your brain fool you. Take a good look at your life, at how your addiction started, and at how it has progressed to today. Addiction is a progressive disease—it only gets worse over time. There is some truth to the saying that the road of addiction leads to one of three things—jail, hospital, or death—for those who continue to addict. As you look to the future, realize that although the road of recovery leads to healing, the road of addiction leads to hell.

What damage have you already suffered? Have you spent a lot of money on painkillers? Have you spent your valuable time trying to get painkillers? Have you tried to hide your addiction from others, throwing you into a disconnected life of secrecy and inauthenticity? Have you been arrested? Have you needed more and more painkillers over time to get the same effect? Have you overdosed on painkillers? Have you restricted your relationships as you have devoted more time to your addiction? Have you given up things you used to enjoy doing? If these things have not yet happened to you, you can be sure that they will with time. Even if your addiction does not take your life, it will take away all the good in your life and leave you and those who love you with only pain.

You may feel that you have no other option. Feeling helpless and hopeless is part of addiction. You may feel that you have no choice but to continue taking painkillers. You may have 100 reasons why you cannot stop. Be very clear with yourself, however, that you do have a choice. You can always choose recovery. There is hope. There is a better way. No matter how bad your pain, there is a solution other than addiction. No matter how severe your cravings, there is a way through them. No matter how intense your withdrawal symptoms, you can survive. No matter how bleak your life has become, there can always be healing and repair. You, too, can heal from your addiction, just as millions have done.

Be clear-eyed and see the truth. Addiction is a progressive disease. Life does not get better if you continue to addict. It only gets worse. You are caught in a brain vortex that is swirling downward into misery and destruction. The simple truth is that if you stop addicting and work on your recovery, your life will eventually get better.

11. Addiction is a chronic disease that can have recurrences.

Addiction is similar in many ways to other chronic medical illnesses, such as diabetes, asthma, and congestive heart failure. People can bring all of these illnesses into remission with good self-care and treatment. The same is true of addiction. With good treatment and good self-care, you can bring your addiction into remission.

Many people with other chronic diseases have flare-ups of their disease. A person with diabetes, for example, may experience high blood sugar if they get an infection, or if they eat too many carbohydrates. A person with congestive heart failure may experience a loss of heart function if they gain too much weight, let their blood pressure get too high, or eat too much salt. All these chronic diseases have conditions that trigger recurrences of illness.

Similarly, people with addiction also experience conditions that can trigger readdicting. Triggers can be internal or external. In all cases, pain is at the root of all triggers, even if it is just the pain of cravings.

Let's examine such triggers. External triggers can be people, places, and situations outside of you. They include seeing painkillers, drug paraphernalia, drug dealers, people you used drugs with, neighborhoods where you got your supply, and places where you addicted. Stressful situations can also trigger readdiction—stress is painful.

As part of your recovery, you will need to identify all the people, places, and situations that trigger you. You will then need to remove these triggers as much as possible. Plan to remove yourself from triggers when they do arise.

Internal triggers are painful, negative emotional states. They can include feeling stressed, angry, anxious, worried, hopeless, envious, lonely, or bored. Shame is also a big trigger for cravings to addict. Physical pain and fatigue are also triggers. In all cases, there is some way that you are not right with Life, either physically, emotionally, or spiritually.

You will need to learn to stay positive and grateful when negativity arises. Learn to soothe yourself and to get support. Make it a rule to not isolate yourself. Talk things out with someone. Get emotional support though a support system you develop.

Don't make negative thoughts and feelings your enemy. Label them, say "thank you," for them, and inquire into the roots of your negativity. Then correct your negative thinking and attitude with acceptance and unconditional self-reverence. Use your support system to resolve your pain and get back on a positive track.

You will also need to develop your craving management skills for when you are triggered. I will teach you ways to manage your cravings in a later lesson. Just know that with practice, you can learn to manage your cravings when you are triggered.

With good self-care, good treatment, and support, you can manage triggers and prevent flare-ups of your addiction. Good recovery is the practice of preventing the pain that triggers readdicting, along with skillful pain management when pain does arise, including the pain of the cravings that you will experience.

Although readdiction is painful, it can actually be the greatest of gifts if you embrace readdiction as an opportunity to learn and grow. Work to prevent flare-ups of your addiction, but don't give up or beat yourself up if they occur. Instead, ask for help, get back up on your feet, recommit to your recovery, and persevere. Make failures your friends. With practice, you will develop your recovery skills to prevent episodes of readdiction. Never give up hope!

12. You will always have a vulnerability to painkillers.

If you have an addiction to painkillers, you will be vulnerable to addiction to painkillers for the rest of your life. Why is this? It is because painkillers likely caused permanent changes to your brain. They permanently turned off the part of the brain that controls cravings. The drugs also caused changes to the shape and structure of some of your brain cells called "neurons." We think these changes make you more vulnerable to addiction.

People say addiction is like turning a cucumber into a pickle. While addiction may be reversible for some people, for many it appears to not be reversible. I hear stories all the time of people who stopped using painkillers for many years and then started using them again, perhaps after an operation or injury. When they started using them again, their addiction began again.

After you get off painkillers for a while, your brain may play a trick on you. That trick is called "complacency." Complacency means thinking you are safe when you are not. Your brain will tell you, "I'm doing great. I'm past that addiction. Things are different now. I can use painkillers now and I will be fine."

If you ever have complacency thoughts like these, know that you are in trouble. You should forever have a healthy fear of painkillers. I have seen countless patients over the years fall right back into addicting when they became complacent. That is why it is said, "Complacency kills." Protect your recovery with eternal vigilance.

You will likely have times in the future when you are in severe pain. You may injure yourself in an accident, or you may need surgery. If these things happen, you will need to be very careful. You should avoid using narcotic painkillers if at all possible. If you must take narcotics for severe pain, you should do so for as short a time as possible and under close supervision, with someone you trust holding onto your painkiller prescription. If you are in the hospital, work with your doctor to be discharged without narcotics. Instead, take non-narcotic pain relievers.

Fentanyl: A Deadly Street Drug

The synthetic painkiller fentanyl is 50 times stronger than heroin and 100 times stronger than morphine. The equivalent of five grains of table salt can kill the average adult.

In hospitals, fentanyl may be injected, delivered as a patch for absorption into the body, or it may be given as a lozenge or lollipop. On the streets, it may be laced into heroin, marijuana, or cocaine to enhance potency.

Other illegal forms include powder, a piece of blotter paper placed under the tongue, or pills. It is often pressed into counterfeit pills that look like legitimate painkillers, and buyers may have no idea the pills contain fentanyl. The illegal drugs are often shipped through the U.S. mail from China or Mexico.

—Center for Disease Control and Prevention

If you must take painkillers, prepare yourself. You may re-experience cravings along with strong urges to take more painkillers. If this happens, you will need to practice your craving management techniques and ask for lots of help to not fall back into your addiction. Make sure you stay connected to your recovery supports—people who can help you manage your cravings.

If you suffer from chronic pain, resist the urge to use addictive painkillers to manage your pain. We now know we can treat chronic non-cancer pain equally well with non-narcotic treatments. If you have chronic pain, schedule an appointment with a pain management specialist about non-addictive treatments. You don't have to suffer from chronic pain. For many, addiction is a chronic disease with periods of remission and recurrences, or flare-ups, of addicting. Know that after you develop an addiction to painkillers you will be vulnerable to recurrences of addicting. You likely will need to avoid taking painkillers, take good care of yourself, and work on your recovery for the rest of your life. You will need to tend to your recovery, just as you would tend to a garden, to protect yourself from your vulnerability to readdicting.

13. Physical dependence on a drug is different from addiction to a drug.

There is a difference between physical dependence on opioids and being addicted to opioids. Let's explore physical dependence in more detail to understand how it is different from addiction.

Let's take coffee as an example for comparison. Do you drink coffee? If you do, you probably notice that you need that first cup in the morning to get going. If you don't have your coffee, you feel sluggish. If you don't drink coffee, you might experience withdrawal symptoms as the day goes on such as headaches. If this happens to you, then you are physiologically dependent on caffeine. You need caffeine to feel normal, and you go into "withdrawal" if you do not have it.

If you don't feel craving to have more and more coffee after your usual intake of coffee from day to day, then you likely are just physically dependent on coffee. You are dependent on coffee, but you are not addicted to coffee. Similarly, many people are dependent upon painkillers, but they are not addicted to them. Addiction is different from physical dependence.

As we discussed in the previous lesson, our brains like to stay in neutral. After drinking coffee for a while, our brains adapt to having caffeine. This becomes the "new normal" for our brains, and the initial strong stimulation of caffeine fades a bit as our brains get used to caffeine.

Another way of thinking about how the brain changes is what is called "habituation," which means to get used to something—it becomes a habit. After a period of novelty, our brains habituate, or get used to, the way things are. If you were to go on a roller coaster, it would be fun the first ride or two. But after 100 rides, you would probably not enjoy it as much. You would have habituated to roller coasters.

Why do we habituate, or get used to things? Again, the brain seems to like to stay in neutral. It is not in our nature to experience intense joy or ecstasy all the time. By staying in neutral, the brain sets us up to experience intermittent rewards for intermittently rewarding experiences. If we were to have Thanksgiving dinner every day, turkey and stuffing would soon get old for most of us. Habituation seems to prompt us to seek out variety in our diet and to introduce a certain amount of novelty into our lives.

So what is the difference between physical dependence and drug addiction? The difference is that with addiction, there are cravings and compulsions to take more and more of a drug. With addiction, you spiral out of control. You continue to compulsively take painkillers to feel better even though they are destroying your life. Addiction is a compulsion to achieve short-term gain despite long-term pain. Addiction is compulsive "good-now bad-later behavior."

If you are physically dependent upon painkillers, you are not addicted. Like with coffee, you need to take painkillers to feel okay and to avoid feeling the pain of withdrawal. But you don't feel a need to take more and more of them in a way that makes you feel out of control. You don't feel the craving to take more to attempt to feel even better. You don't experience any adverse consequences of being addicted to painkillers— consequences such as loss of jobs, loss of relationships, and financial problems.

Just as people can be dependent on a substance without being addicted, the opposite is true as well. You can be addicted without being dependent. A good example of this would be some people who have an addiction to cocaine or methamphetamine. After heavy use for a day or two, they may crash for a day and then be back to feeling normal. Then, perhaps a week or two later, the cravings for cocaine or methamphetamine come creeping back into their brains. Along with cravings, they feel compulsions to addict and a loss of control, and the cycle of addiction recurs. Another example is someone who binge drinks once a week; they are addicted but not dependent.

If you have an addiction to painkillers, you likely have both physiological dependence and addiction. If you stop using painkillers suddenly, you will likely feel both the pain of withdrawal along with intense cravings and compulsions to take painkillers. That is why most people suffering from opioid use disorder need detoxification to help their brains adapt back to not having opioids in their system.

If you have only a physical dependence on painkillers, then you might be able to undergo a slow tapering off of them and not need further addiction treatment. If you suffer from addiction, however, you will likely benefit from addiction treatment to recover.

PART II
What You Need to Know about Treatment

14. There is hope—treatment works.

Do you feel like your addiction is hopeless? Do you feel that your life is hopeless? If so, you are not alone. Almost everyone feels both hopeless and ashamed because of their addiction. It is discouraging and demoralizing to be caught up in addiction, compulsively using painkillers even when you desperately want to stop—you realize that you are repeatedly harming yourself and others along the way.

The biggest problem I see is some people's belief that they will never be able to live a happy life without painkillers. Is that how you feel? If so, you probably feel that life on life's terms is unbearable. You may not believe that it is possible to have a joyful life without painkillers. You may have even stopped painkillers for a while and found that life was bleak or even miserable. You may feel that living a fulfilling life is impossible for you. You may feel that the gratification of getting high is your only option. You may feel that the urge to addict is just too great. You may feel that while recovery may be possible for others, it is just not an option for you.

You may suffer from trauma, psychiatric illness, or medical illness. You may have a history of mistakes and failures that leave you feeling you are a hopeless loser. You may feel you are beyond hope and beyond repair.

If this is the case for you, know this: treatment works if it is good treatment and you do the work required to heal and realize a joyful life. You will not recover if you expect someone to fix you. But you will recover if you humbly stick to treatment and do the work of recovery. You are right that life is difficult. It is true that it can take a lot of work, treatment, and practice to realize a joyful life without painkillers. Healing is hard work, but it is possible. If you look around you, you will see that there are many people who managed to recover through a combination of treatment, the support of others, and their own hard work. If they can do it, so can you. It takes the willingness to get treatment and do the work. With hope and humility—having a modest opinion of yourself rather than an inflated sense of yourself—you can free yourself from this addiction.

Although recovery is hard work, it is well worth the effort. One pound of joy is far more valuable than one hundred pounds of narcotic gratification. No matter how joyless you feel now, know that you will eventually experience joy if you do the work outlined in this book and get the treatment you need.

Although you may not be able to stop on your own, you need to know that your addiction can go into remission with proper treatment. Invariably, those who stick with their treatment and do the work of recovery do well. As I will discuss in a later lesson, powerful medications now exist that either take away cravings or protect you from addiction if you do fall back into using painkillers. Effective therapy and recovery supports exist almost everywhere to help you.

The field of addictions treatment is rapidly evolving lifesaving evidence-based treatments. You may feel hopeless, but this feeling is not reality. The reality is that there is great hope for you!

To find a good treatment center, you can do an Internet search for "addiction treatment centers near me." You might also ask your primary care physician or another health care provider for a referral. As a last resort, you can go to your nearest emergency room, where the staff can help stabilize your withdrawal symptoms if necessary and refer you to a treatment program.

Good addictions treatment does not have to be at a high-end residential treatment center. If you have a safe and supportive recovery environment, you can succeed with outpatient treatment, even in a doctor's office.

In many treatment centers, the medical professionals adhere to the following principles:

- *Commitment to integrity and excellence:* Make sure your provider is committed to integrity and excellence. The provider should assess patient satisfaction and outcomes. If a treatment center is residential, the staff should teach patients how to live a healthful lifestyle by modeling it in their programs.

- *Accessible:* You should have relatively fast access to treatment, especially if you are in withdrawal.

- *Safe, compassionate, and respectful:* Staff should create a climate of respect, safety, and trust. Staff should not confront or demean patients. Staff should be kind, firm, and flexible. Staff should respect your confidentiality, including in group treatment. Drug testing should be used only to monitor recovery status, and never in a punitive way.

- *Patient-centered and responsive:* Staff should help you decide on how you wish to pursue recovery, as everyone's path is unique. Staff should match treatment to your individual needs and preferences.

- *Patient-empowering:* The program should empower you to manage your own recovery with the help of others and recognize that you will need a "Greater Power" than yourself to help empower you in your recovery.

- *Recovery- and discovery-oriented:* While all treatment programs will provide you an abstinence-based approach to recovery, they should also honor your wish to try to find a way to reduce the harm of your addiction if that is what you want. If you are not sure what you want, the treatment program should offer to help you figure out what is best for you.

- *Total recovery-oriented:* A good treatment program will encourage you to not harm yourself in any way by addicting. They should offer you help to become free of all addictions. They should address the six foundations of recovery: motivation, coping with

27

cravings, managing emotions, nurturing relationships, creating a balanced lifestyle, and finding purpose in life. In balancing work, love, and play, they should provide assistance as needed with an exercise plan, a personal recreation plan, education on healthful nutrition, and assistance with developing a daily spiritual practice.

- *Comprehensive and integrated:* The best programs will provide or arrange for integrated medical, psychiatric, and psychological treatment for all psychological issues, not just your addiction. They should arrange for specialty treatment for issues such as gender issues and eating disorders. They should have a capacity to address trauma.

- *Recovery support-oriented:* Your treatment provider should be there for you over the long run, ready and able to help you with flare-ups of readdiction. Good programs will support you beyond detox and help you to develop a stable recovery.

- *Community- and family-oriented:* Your provider should provide case management services and family therapy. They should collaborate with your other treatment providers.

- *Evidence-based care:* Your provider should provide care that has been shown to be effective in the research on treatment. This includes family therapy, couples therapy, individual therapy, emotional trauma therapy, group therapy, and helpful support groups.

- *Committed to long-term care and recovery:* Your provider should recognize that recovery is a lifelong process. An ideal program will be there for you for the three to five years that it takes most people to establish a stable recovery, and even longer if that is what you need. A good program will even have an alumni program to support you over the years to come.

Not all treatment programs are the same. Look for treatment programs that have board-certified or licensed clinicians with specialty training in addictions treatment. Also look for programs that are accredited by the Joint Commission on Accreditation of Healthcare Organizations (JCAHO).

A word about health insurance. If you have health insurance, they most likely will pay for your treatment. Insurance payers certify benefits according to "medical necessity" criteria. What this means is that they will pay for the services you need at the level of care you need, but will not pay for care that they feel is more than you need. They will generally pay for residential treatment if you need twenty-four-hour professional support and supervision. If you are high functioning and have a safe, sober, and supportive place to stay, your insurance company may pay only for intensive outpatient care. Your treatment provider will generally work with your insurance company to get approval for the level of care that is right for you.

15. To begin treatment, you need medical detoxification to get off painkillers.

Good treatment will ease the pain of withdrawal. As you probably know, withdrawal from opioids is miserable. It is like having a very bad case of the flu. Early opioid withdrawal symptoms include:

- Muscle aches
- Restlessness
- Anxiety
- Eyes tearing up
- Runny nose
- Sweating
- Insomnia
- Yawning

As withdrawal progresses, you will likely experience:

- Diarrhea
- Abdominal cramping
- Goose bumps
- Nausea and vomiting
- Dilated pupils

- Rapid heartbeat
- High blood pressure

You may have experienced some of these symptoms. After you're in treatment, withdrawal usually starts getting better after about three days. Most symptoms go away after about a week. Although withdrawal can seem unbearable, you should know that it is not life threatening. Also, remember that opioid withdrawal is temporary. As it is often said, with opioid addiction, sometimes you have to go through "hell" (withdrawal) to get to "heaven" (recovery).

Medical detoxification—the medically supervised process for stopping opioid use—can take place in either a residential treatment setting or in an outpatient setting. Detoxification usually includes a physical exam or at least a review of your overall health prior to detoxification.

Let's talk about the two most common ways of detoxing off painkillers. One way is to transition to the medication called buprenorphine. It is sold under several brand names; Suboxone is one of the common brands. This drug is an opioid-like medication that partially stimulates the part of the brain involved in your addiction; buprenorphine takes away cravings and withdrawal symptoms without creating a "high."

One of the main benefits of buprenorphine is that you don't have to go through much withdrawal. If you're going to take buprenorphine, you will begin with a one-day washout—to get opioids out of your system. You need to be in moderate withdrawal before you can start buprenorphine; if you take buprenorphine when you have opioids in your system, the buprenorphine can throw you into severe withdrawal. During this washout time, your prescriber will likely give you comfort medications as needed for withdrawal symptoms. These include medications for fever, chills, headache, muscle pain, nausea, abdominal cramps, muscle spasms, diarrhea, insomnia, and anxiety.

You will likely begin to feel normal after just a few days after starting buprenorphine. See the lesson on medications to help you stay sober to learn more about buprenorphine.

A second way to get off painkillers is to slowly taper off opioids with another opioid while taking different comfort medications for withdrawal symptoms. If you taper off opioids, your prescriber will give you tapering doses of another opioid—often methadone or tramadol—to ease you off of opioids. Methadone is a long-acting opioid painkiller that provides a smooth, gradual reduction of opioid levels in your blood over several days. Methadone reduces the severity of withdrawal symptoms and helps to ease you off of opioids. Another drug, tramadol, is a relatively weak opioid-like medication that also reduces withdrawal symptoms. Tramadol also helps to ease you off of opioids. The process of tapering off opioids usually takes about five to eight days. This tapering method is best if you are planning to stay sober without medications (which is not recommended), or if your prescriber is planning to prescribe the drug naltrexone. This drug completely blocks your brain's opioid receptors so that painkillers won't work—you get no effect from them. Naltrexone protects you from readdicting as long as you continue to take it. (I will talk more about naltrexone in the lesson on medications to help you stay sober.)

If I am transitioning a patient onto naltrexone to help them stay sober, I like to prescribe a one-day dose of buprenorphine on day two of withdrawal to ease withdrawal symptoms. I prescribe comfort medications, and then slowly give increasing doses of naltrexone starting on day four. With this protocol, most patients can receive a long-acting injection of naltrexone on day eight.

Whether you transition to buprenorphine or taper off opioids, your prescriber will likely give you comfort medications to reduce your withdrawal symptoms. See the table on page 32 that lists withdrawal symptoms and the medications your prescriber may give you to treat these symptoms.

After you have completed your medical detoxification and are feeling better, you will be facing the circumstances that addiction has visited upon your life. You may need a place to live or you may need a job. You may need to secure a safe and supportive living situation that will promote your recovery. You may have a toxic network of relationships with others who are caught up in addiction. Many of your family and friends may be hurt and even angry over the ways you have treated them.

Medications to Treat Withdrawal Symptoms

Withdrawal Symptom	Medication
Fever, chills, sweating	Clonidine, lofexidine
Muscle spasms	Methocarbamol
Pain	Ibuprofen, acetaminophen, naproxen
Abdominal cramps	Dicyclomine
Nausea	Ondansetron, prochlorperazine
Insomnia	Zolpidem, trazodone
Anxiety	Lorazepam, clonazepam
Restless legs	Ropinrole, pramipexole

It may take some time to create a supportive recovery environment, develop healthy, sober relationships, and secure meaningful, rewarding work. It will also take some time to heal your damaged relationships. You will need to persist with your treatment while you work on rebuilding your life and healing the damage caused by your addiction. Have faith that if you just persevere and give it time, your treatment will help you to create a joyful life.

Although I have seen a few patients over the years who have kicked their opioid habit on their own, most people need help. If you are dependent on narcotics, you will likely need professional help in the form of medical detoxification to get off of them.

16. Even after getting through withdrawal, you may experience distress; however, this distress is treatable.

Getting sober can be an incredible relief. It can also be painful, as you wake up and begin to see things more clearly. You may experience sadness, grief, and shame. Expect these feelings and welcome them as a normal and natural response to your addiction. You may experience three different types of distress after withdrawal:

- The distress of Post-Acute Withdrawal Syndrome (PAWS)
- The distress of facing and dealing with the damage your addiction caused to you and your loved ones

- The emotional or physical distress of any preexisting trauma, neglect, psychiatric conditions, or medical conditions that you endured prior to and along with your addiction.

Let's first talk about PAWS. Unless you go on buprenorphine or methadone, you may continue to feel poorly with symptoms of what's called Post-Acute Withdrawal Syndrome (PAWS). These symptoms may include depression, mood swings, anxiety, irritability, fatigue, agitation, or insomnia. These low-grade, longer-term post-withdrawal symptoms can last for weeks to months. If you have these symptoms, take heart, for they almost always go away. Also, your prescriber and your therapist can help treat them. I recommend the following for managing PAWS:

- Exercise
- Adequate sleep
- Good nutrition
- Rest
- The practice of mindful acceptance of distress
- Distraction with relaxing and fun activities
- Music
- Yoga, acupuncture, and massage

In addition, I also sometimes treat PAWS with medications, especially for insomnia. Antidepressants and mood stabilizers may sometimes help. I avoid benzodiazepines for anxiety, because they are addictive and may create an additional problem.

In rare cases, PAWS can last a long time. If that is the case for you, you may want to consider going on buprenorphine. It takes away PAWS completely. It may also have an antidepressant effect for some. Some people just don't ever feel right after they come off opioids. For some, the use of opioids seems to change the brain, leaving them with what may be an "endorphin deficit disorder." Endorphins are the opioid-like "messengers" in your brain that reduce pain and create a sense of well-being.

Talk out your feelings and get help from your recovery supports. You can also talk to your prescriber about medications to help treat PAWS. Reassure yourself that PAWS almost always goes away with time as your brain heals.

Suboxone: Find a Physician

Physicians must receive special training to prescribe Suboxone (buprenorphine), the drug used to treat opioid addiction. To find a physician in your area, visit: www.suboxone.com.

The second type of pain is the emotional pain from the damage your addiction has done to your life and the lives of those around you. Addiction is traumatic. Once you get sober, you will need to go about the work of rebuilding your life and repairing your relationships. You may experience shame, remorse, and guilt. Be careful, because these emotions can take you right back into addiction. You will need to move beyond shame, remorse, and guilt with acceptance, forgiveness, and the other techniques I talked about in the previous lesson on shame.

Have faith during the early part of your recovery that things will slowly get better, one day at at time. Practice patience and perseverance. Give yourself time to repair and rebuild your life. It may take several months or even years. If you stay sober and do the work, things WILL slowly get better!

You will need to make amends to the people you have hurt. You may even need to make restitution. See the lesson on the importance of connections for more information on repairing relationships.

The third type of pain you may experience when you get sober is emotional or physical pain that you had before you developed opioid addiction. If you're like most people, you fell into addiction through a combination of emotional or physical pain and a genetic vulnerability to addiction.

If your pain is primarily physical, seek out comprehensive non-narcotic pain management treatment from a team of pain management specialists. Options include non-narcotic medications, acupuncture, massage, physical therapy, and pain psychotherapy. Research shows that most people can get just as good or even better pain management without narcotics.

If you had emotional pain prior to your addiction due to trauma, neglect, or psychiatric illness, it may have been subtle, such as a vague sense of unease, boredom, unworthiness, or restlessness. Or, your emotional pain may have been severe, such as intense anger, agitation, painful memories, emptiness, depression, or anxiety. You may have experienced all these emotions and more. Since we all want to feel good and not feel bad, it is natural and understandable if you used painkillers to numb either physical or emotional pain.

When you are sober, you will need to learn to resolve the preexisting pain of trauma, neglect, and psychiatric illness skillfully and wisely—with love—instead of numbing it with narcotic pleasure. Recovery is about living life on Life's terms and learning to skillfully manage your pain. I've devoted much of this book to discussing love-based ways of resolving emotional pain and enhancing your joy. The following is a brief summary of what you will need to do in your early recovery once you get sober.

There are several ways to resolve emotional pain with love:

- *Practice a spiritual attitude of unconditional appreciation of all experience, including pain.* Remind yourself that this moment is sacred and can only be exactly as it is. Ask yourself what your pain is trying to teach you. Pain is a stern but crucial messenger that things are not right. Be humble, acceptant, and open to your pain. Let your pain teach you. When you accept and even welcome your pain, suffering diminishes. This takes effort and practice. Be patient and give this practice time to work.

- *Face and embrace your pain, rather than run from it.* Pain that you run away from will haunt you until you face and address it. When you face your pain, you position yourself to act to resolve it.

- *Talk out your pain with others. Remember to never hurt alone.* Regulate your emotions by accessing the support of others. Let others help you to endure, persevere, and problem-solve ways to reduce your pain. Remember that no one does recovery alone. Surround yourself with the love of others.

- *Get psychiatric and medical treatment as needed to dimminish your distress.*

- *Nurture and soothe yourself.* Do things that are fun, relaxing, and calming. Spend time in nature, exercise, treat yourself to a bath or a massage, listen to music, read something positive and inspiring, or do one of a thousand other things that might help you feel better.

- *Take perspective.* Note that all things are impermanent. Your pain will eventually pass as long as you keep doing the next right thing with love and integrity.

One secret to a long, stable, and joyful life is skillful pain management. Up until now you've numbed pain with pleasure and fell into the trap of addiction. Now make the practice of managing pain with love one of your core recovery practices. The rest of this book will give you further guidance in the art of pain management in recovery.

17. Residential treatment is a live-in health care facility that provides treatment for substance abuse.
    Residental treatment provides a home-like environment where you can receive twenty-four hour clinical supervision and support. Lengths of stay in a residential setting vary from a few days to a few weeks, depending on how long you need twenty-four-hour professional support, supervision, and clinical care. Residential treatment provides such support, usually with up to daily availability of medical personnel if you are undergoing detoxification. A medical provider may need to see you as frequently as daily if you are detoxing; during these frequent visits, your prescriber can adjust your detox medications if needed.
    Residential care is appropriate if you are emotionally unstable and need twenty-four-hour structure and support to function, stay safe, and stay sober. Residential care may also be appropriate if you are new to recovery or have several other issues other than your addiction; this might include such things as other psychiatric problems or medical issues. A residential

treatment center may be right for you until you are stabilized and are feeling well and safe enough to continue treatment on an outpatient basis.

Most residential programs have about four hours of group therapy a day. In some treatment facilities, group treatment programs focus on various recovery issues such as:

- Managing cravings and triggers
- The effects of addiction on the brain
- Managing emotional and physical pain
- Healing trauma and neglect
- Healthy relationships with family members and others
- Self-care skills
- Healthy lifestyles
- Stress management
- Spirituality/love in recovery
- Orientation to recovery and treatment
- Mutual help groups
- Recovery mentors and supports
- Cultivating wisdom and clarity

Most programs will also have "process group therapy." This type of group therapy is intended to help individuals better understand themselves and their relationships so that they can make healthier choices based on greater insights about themselves.

At many treatment facilities, clients meet weekly with a therapist and with an alcohol and drug counselor. The therapist helps you develop an understanding of your situation and constructs a treatment plan with you. They see you both individually and with your family, helping your family learn how to best support you in your recovery. The Alcohol and Drug counselor helps you learn to manage triggers and cravings and to develop a readdiction prevention plan.

A good residential program will promote healthy living. They will schedule time, for example, for morning prayer or meditation and for exercise. They will also help you to practice recovery skills such as how to manage cravings and stress.

Electrical Stimulation to Treat Withdrawal

Another detox option does not involve medications. It is a device called an "auricular stimulator," and it lessens withdrawal symptoms. Your provider will tape this small electronic device behind your ear and attach four electrodes to different parts of your ear. The device delivers repeated pulses of electricity to several points on the ear for about five days; it is similar to acupuncture. I have used this device on a number of patients and have seen dramatic effects. The auricular stimulator can reduce or even eliminate the need for comfort medications.

18. You can also receive addiction treatment in outpatient settings.

As the name suggests, outpatient treatment does not involve residing at a treatment center. Instead, you live at home during your treatment. With outpatient treatment, you also go through detoxification to lessen the discomfort of withdrawal. So, if you are fairly stable emotionally and have a safe and supportive home environment, you may be able to begin the drug buprenorphine as part of outpatient treatment.

Your provider will likely offer you medications to help you stay sober. Using such medications during treatment leads to six to eight times higher rates of recovery than for people who attempt to recover without medications. See the lesson on medications to help you stay sober for more information.

Many patients live in toxic recovery environments. They may not need residential treatment, but in order to recover, they need a safe, supportive, low-stress environment. If you don't have a safe and supportive home environment, your provider may help arrange for a home-like setting, such as a "sober home," for you to live while you receive outpatient treatment.

There are tens of thousands of sober homes around the nation. Often, you can stay in a sober home, paying on a month-to-month basis. Meals are usually provided. A house manager looks after the home and the residents. They do urine drug screenings to ensure sobriety. Some sober homes will hold recovery meetings on the premises. The house manager is usually someone who is also in recovery.

Many treatment centers have their own sober homes where patients can stay while they attend partial hospital or intensive outpatient treatment. If you should choose to stay in a sober home, make sure the home has strong management and is operated ethically.

Your treatment needs determine which level of outpatient care you need. There are three levels of outpatient care:

- *Partial hospital level of care,* which can be up to six to eight hours of treatment five or more days a week.

- *Intensive outpatient care,* which is usually about three hours a day, two to five days a week.

- *Regular (low intensity) outpatient,* which is usually one hour one to two days a week.

If you are new to recovery, are having a lot of cravings, are feeling emotionally unstable, or lack any recovery supports, then partial hospital care may be the best starting place for you. If you are feeling stable and have a good emotional support system, you may only need to see a therapist in private practice along with a doctor, who can treat your withdrawal symptoms with medication.

You may step down from a higher intensity of treatment to a lower level over time. Many people go from residential to partial hospital to intensive outpatient treatment to regular outpatient treatment. Your partial hospital or intensive outpatient care should also have a therapist who can work with you and your family.

Partial hospital and intensive outpatient care generally last from one to four weeks, depending on your treatment needs and what your insurance will pay. Most people in outpatient treatment benefit from three to five years of treatment, though treatment may even be lifelong if you have one or more serious and persistent psychiatric conditions or if you are on medication maintenance treatment.

Looking for a Treatment Center?

Substance Abuse and Mental Health Services Administration (SAMHSA) offers an online treatment facility locator at: www.findtreatment.samhsa. gov. The locator includes more than 12,000 addiction treatment programs, including residential treatment centers, outpatient treatment programs, and hospital inpatient programs for drug addiction and alcoholism.

No matter what level of care you receive, you will need a supportive recovery environment. If you don't have a supportive home environment that is safe, stable, sober, and supervised, then you may need to live in a sober living home while you are getting outpatient treatment. If you need long-term support while working on your recovery and other life skills, then you might need to live in a longer-term sober home or group home.

Outpatient care enables you to begin to develop the outside recovery routines and supports you will need to succeed in your recovery. I especially recommend intensive outpatient care in the community where you will be living, so that you can set up your long-term recovery supports and routines, including support group meetings.

Your treatment provider should provide you the level of care according to your needs, which will change over time. Feel comfortable to talk with your provider about the levels of care that are best for you.

19. Medications can help you stay sober.

As you know, opioid addiction can cause severe cravings and compulsions to addict. Even the most strong-willed and skillful person can succumb to the power of the disease despite their best intentions. This is why only about 10 to 20 percent of people with opioid use disorder manage to stay sober longer than a year after their detoxification treatment without a medication to help them stay sober. We must be humble in the face of the powerful neurobiological illness called "addiction."

For this reason, you should strongly consider going on a medication to help you stay sober.

Some people frown on medications, mistakenly believing that you are "not sober" if you are on medications. Disregard these opinions. They are wrong. If you are not addicting, you are sober. Ironically, many of these people who say they are "clean and sober" and pass judgment on people who are on medications are actively addicting and destroying themselves with cigarettes. As a general life rule, don't let the judgments of others sway you from doing what is best for you.

There are primarily three medications available that help you stay sober:

- *Methadone*—a synthetic opioid prescribed for moderate to severe pain. Prescribers also use it to treat opiate addictions.

- *Naltrexone*—a medication used to treat alcohol or opioid dependence. Sold under the brand names ReVia, Vivitrol, and others.

- *Buprenorphine*—is an opioid-like medication used to treat opioid addiction and pain. It is sold under the brand name Suboxone and others.

Methadone is the most effective drug for staying sober, with abstinence rates as high as 80 percent or more. Methadone is itself a narcotic and a painkiller. If you are under medical care, methadone can serve as a safe substitute for the painkillers you are using.

There are some drawbacks to methadone maintenance treatment. You must go to a licensed methadone maintenance clinic to receive this treatment. This can be a problem if there is no methadone maintenance clinic near you. Treatment can also be inconvenient due to the need to go to the clinic every day for your dose.

Methadone can make you feel apathetic. It can also cause constipation, which is generally manageable. Methadone is also somewhat more risky than naltrexone and buprenorphine. If you take other painkillers, alcohol, or sedatives with methadone, you may put yourself at risk of overdose and death. Every year a small number of people on methadone maintenance die from accidental or intentional overdoses.

Methadone can also rarely cause your heart to stop beating. Your methadone maintenance provider will likely obtain an EKG to check your heart rhythm during your treatment. They will also check to make sure methadone is safe to take with your other medications.

Another drug, naltrexone, also helps you stay sober. This drug blocks opioids from binding to the brain's opioid receptors—the ones involved in opioid addiction. Naltrexone is very helpful in protecting you from a negative state of mind and the cravings that drive readdiction. It reduces cravings, helps to make your life manageable, and enables you to turn your attention to the work of recovery. As long as you are on naltrexone, you are virtually 100 percent protected from readdicting.

Opioids must be out of your system before you can take naltrexone. This is because if you have opioids in your system when you take naltrexone, naltrexone will block your opioid receptors and throw you into severe withdrawal. Because of this, your provider will only give you naltrexone after you have tapered off opioids. Keep in mind that tapering off of opioids will cause you to experience withdrawal symptoms, which your provider will need to treat with various comfort medications.

Another benefit of naltrexone is that when you are ready to come off it, which is usually in about three years for many people, you can just stop the medication. You won't experience any withdrawal symptoms as you do when you come off buprenorphine.

If you decide to go onto naltrexone, you may experience PAWS. If so, you will need to work with your provider to get treatment for the symptoms of PAWS as discussed in a previous lesson.

Naltrexone comes in pill form and as a long-acting injectable form (Vivitrol) that you can receive once every four weeks so that you are protected as long as you keep getting your shots every month. You may also have the option of receiving a naltrexone implant under your skin that can last up to four to six months. You will need to take naltrexone orally for at least a week or two to make sure you tolerate it before going on injectable shots or receiving the implant.

In rare cases, Naltrexone causes liver inflammation, so you will want to be mindful of right upper abdominal tenderness, fatigue, or just feeling generally ill. Naltrexone can also cause nausea and headaches, and sometimes depression. Usually, these side effects go away after a week or two.

Of all the drug treatments for staying sober off opioids, naltrexone may be the best option for you, even though it is not quite as effective as methadone. There is no physical dependence, and naltrexone protects you nearly 100 percent from readdicting as long as you take it. The problem with naltrexone is that you have to go through withdrawal and be off all opioids before you can take it. Some people find withdrawal unbearable, even with good treatment. For them, either methadone or buprenorphine may be better options.

Buprenorphine is the third medication option for staying sober. Buprenorphine, like methadone, also stimulates brain opioid receptors, but only partially. The drug takes away withdrawal symptoms and cravings for most people without creating a "high."

Buprenorphine is well tolerated—most people feel normal while taking it. It has minimal side effects. It is also more convenient than methadone, because you can fill a prescription and take it at home; you don't have to go to a clinic every day for your dose. After you are stable in your recovery, your prescriber may only see you once a month.

One drawback of buprenorphine is that it can be difficult to come off of. You will experience withdrawal symptoms. For some people, withdrawal off of buprenorphine is worse than withdrawing from painkillers. For this reason, some people stay on buprenorphine for years or even for life. For many people, this is not a problem, for the benefits of buprenorphine far outweigh the minimal cost and inconvenience of treatment.

Another drawback of buprenorphine is that it can make you feel so normal that you almost forget you have an addiction and need to do the work of recovery. If you go on medication, you must remain steadfast and committed to doing your recovery work to create a joyful, stable, and fulfilling life. You should not depend solely on medication for your recovery.

If you decide to go on buprenorphine, your prescriber will likely start you on buprenorphine on your second day of withdrawal, as I discussed in the previous lesson on withdrawal. Your prescriber may then see you daily and give you your medications for each day. If you start buprenorphine as an outpatient, your prescriber will require that you reside in a safe and supportive environment. They will also likely require that someone be with you twenty-four hours a day to make sure you are safe and sober, to monitor you, and to administer your medications.

It's important to remember that things will get better. If you can just make it through those really hard first months, it's going to be amazing how much better things will be, especially if you're in the right environment.

John, 36

Stabilizing on buprenorphine usually takes only two to three days. Many prescribers will require that you stay in their office, sometimes for several hours, on the first day you receive buprenorphine. This is so they can administer buprenorphine to you and monitor your response. There are some prescribers, however, who may give you buprenorphine to take at home. They may see you every day for two to three days until your withdrawal symptoms and cravings have gone away.

On the first day of buprenorphine treatment, your prescriber will start your day with a small dose of buprenorphine, generally two milligrams. You will put this medication under your tongue, where it dissolves. Then, you will likely wait one to two hours. Your prescriber will then assess your withdrawal symptoms. If you are still experiencing withdrawal, your physicians will likely give you another two milligram dose of buprenorphine and then reassess you in another two hours.

Most prescribers will continue to dose you every one to two hours until you receive a total of eight to twelve milligrams of buprenorphine or your withdrawal symptoms go away. The next day you will receive the dose you received the first day. You may then receive more buprenorphine if you are still having withdrawal symptoms. Most prescribers will give you up to sixteen to twenty-four milligrams of buprenorphine a day to control your cravings and withdrawal symptoms. After two to four days, you will likely feel good, with little if any withdrawal symptoms or cravings.

Buprenorphine is helpful because it takes away withdrawal symptoms and cravings. You don't have to go through a complete withdrawal process, so you have much less discomfort. Buprenorphine is also very well tolerated, with few side effects. With buprenorphine, you also avoid PAWS.

You should probably go on one of these medications as part of your recovery, unless you and your providers are confident you are the one out of ten who can manage your cravings without medications. Discuss the risks, benefits, pros, and cons of these medications with your prescriber. Remember that people have about a 90 percent chance of going back to painkillers (readdicting) if they are not on methadone, buprenorphine, or naltrexone. Be humble and realistic about the power of your addiction to take over despite your best intentions. Don't let pride or shame get in the way of your doing everything you can to maximize your chances of success, including taking one of these three medications.

20. In choosing a therapist, be sure to select one with training and experience in treating addictions.

How do you choose a good therapist? A good therapist will assess your needs and help you to choose the interventions and services you receive. Unfortunately, the addiction treatment field is full of the erroneous belief that you are not "sober" if you take medications to treat your addiction. Be wary of therapists who make proclamations about what treatment should be with no evidence base to support their beliefs. Make sure your therapist has training and experience in treating addictions. It is even better if they have some sort of certification in addictions treatment.

Good therapists use treatments that have been scientifically proven to be effective. Many therapists use a combination of therapeutic approaches. You are unique, so the best form of treatment for you will also be unique. As you heal and grow, your needs will change over time. Therefore, the nature of your treatment will need to change along the way. Work with a therapist who understands both your needs and preferences and works to provide individualized treatment.

Look for a therapist who can address all your psychiatric needs, not just your addictions. A therapist who can also help you with other issues is better than treatment that is chopped up among several therapists.

The most important thing to look for in a therapist is for someone who makes you feel safe, supported, and understood. I recommend following the "three-session rule." If, after three sessions, you don't feel your therapist is helping you or you don't feel you have a good connection with them, thank them for their service and look for another therapist. You want to find someone who is not only technically competent, but who also has a good heart and is wise. It can take some effort on your part to find someone who is the right match for you. Keep at it until you find someone who can help you.

What kind of ongoing therapy will help you? After you get sober, I suggest you see a therapist for three to five years, or perhaps even longer if necessary. Use ongoing therapy to:

- Create a safe recovery environment.
- Learn to manage cravings and triggers.
- Learn to manage stress.
- Develop healthy relationships.
- Heal from trauma and neglect.
- Manage negative emotional states, such as boredom, lack of meaning, hopelessness, emptiness, anger, anxiety, and loneliness.
- Create a fulfilling and joyful life.

Once you have healed, feel safe and stable in your recovery, and are living a fulfilling and joyful life, you can stop treatment, although you might want to see your therapist periodically for "checkup" appointments.

Whatever you do, work on your recovery in some way every day until the day you die. This might include your spiritual practice, talking to a recovery supports or mentor, and going to mutual help meetings.

46

21. Treatment may include individual therapy, family therapy, and group therapy.

Your treatment may include a variety of treatment types and formats. You will almost certainly benefit from individual therapy at a minimum. Your therapist will help you to maintain your motivation for recovery, to feel better, to manage cravings and triggers, and to develop recovery routines and supports. Your therapist will help you to repair your life, to live life skillfully, and to resolve pain wisely rather than numb it addictively. They will also help you to heal from trauma and from other psychiatric illnesses.

You will also likely benefit from couples or family therapy if you have loved ones involved in your life. Remember that no one recovers alone. You will need your family's support to maximize your chances of success.

There is a special type of family and couples therapy, called "Community Reinforcement and Family Therapy," or "CRAFT," that is effective in helping your loved ones to help you in your recovery. It might be ideal for you to work with a therapist who can both see you individually and also work with your loved ones to teach them CRAFT techniques. CRAFT will help your loved ones to:

- Reward your positive recovery behavior.

- Withdraw rewards when you are addicting, or detach from your negative addiction behavior.

- Provide you with consistent, unconditional emotional support through positive communications.

- Allow you to experience the natural, therapeutic, negative consequences of your addictive and other unskillful behaviors so that you can learn and grow from your pain.

Oftentimes our loved ones don't understand addiction. They want to help you, but they don't know how. They may make you feel ashamed, frustrated, or angry. You will find CRAFT techniques much more helpful than the nagging, pleading, and criticizing you may have experienced from loved ones up until now.

You may also benefit from group therapy. Group therapy can be especially helpful if you have difficulty making close, positive, authentic connections with others. This might be especially true for you if you experienced abuse, neglect, or other trauma growing up. This is because abuse and neglect damage the development of our emotional and relationship capacities.

My shame made me afraid of treatment. I remember seeing my therapist for the first time. I was shaking. I was so scared, but I remember my therapist, saying in a very calm voice, "Okay, Susan, we're going to get through this."

Susan, 38

If you experience difficulties safely loving and being loved, then an outpatient group therapy would be good for you. Under the protection and guidance of the group therapist, you can practice being spontaneous, authentic, and appropriate with your fellow group members. This can be scary and uncomfortable at first. With some courage and the support of your therapist, you can begin to take small risks, sharing your true thoughts and feelings with others. You can slowly learn to be vulnerable. You can learn to acknowledge others as well as let them see the real you.

In good group therapy, hurt feelings, misunderstandings, and misperceptions inevitably arise. It is the job of your therapist to help you and your fellow group members to work through these difficult moments. Such moments are an opportunity for the group to develop greater clarity, understanding, empathy, and compassion for each other. Remember, this group setting is a "safe place," for you to learn—to work through issues while you have a professional therapist there to guide and teach you. This is where the process of emotional healing is strongest, as you develop your relationship capacities. Because we all need each other to get by, good group therapy will help you regulate your painful emotions by accessing the understanding, support, and wisdom of the group. With time and practice, group therapy can help you to take your newfound relational skills and put them into practice in your life.

Talk with your therapist about your needs. You may well benefit from a combination of individual, family, and group treatment. Make sure you get the treatment you need to maximize your chances of success in your recovery.

22. Treatment takes time.

You will need to be patient and persistent. It may take from three to five years of intensive treatment followed by long-term outpatient treatment for you to realize a stable and joyful recovery. Be patient with the process of healing and growth that lies before you. Just as a baby takes nine months to grow before being ready for birth, so you will need time in treatment to heal and grow.

The road of recovery has its ups and downs. There will be times when you will likely feel hopeless and discouraged. There will be times when you will feel like giving up. Know that this is normal. Hang in there with your treatment and persist. You will succeed in your recovery if you endure and persist through the dark times.

If you feel your treatment is not working, talk about this with your therapist. Work to change your treatment if necessary, or look for a new therapist who can better meet your needs. Don't make the mistake of walking away from treatment before you have achieved a stable and joyful life free of addiction.

You may even experience reoccurrences of addiction along the way. If this happens to you, don't give up. Stick with your treatment, learn from your mistakes, and leverage readdiction as an opportunity to grow.

You may decide to continue long-term outpatient treatment for even longer, perhaps for a lifetime. Recovery is a lifelong process of growth and transformation. Your treatment can help you with your growth and healing over a lifetime as well.

The thing that needs to change in recovery is everything. Change requires practice and repetition of new ways of being, seeing, and doing. You will need time to learn and practice new life skills that help you to:

- Manage cravings
- Manage triggers
- Reduce shame and develop a sense of wholeness

- Heal from trauma, psychiatric illnesses, and medical illnesses
- Realize meaning and purpose through your daily activities
- Have fun and savor the joy of existence
- Minimize stress and distress
- Develop safe, loving relationships
- Develop your capacity to experience the Sacred, or the extraordinary in the ordinary

You will need time in treatment with one or more therapists and other recovery supports to develop these life skills. Becoming a master at anything, including the ability to live a joyful life free of addiction, takes thousands of hours of consistent, daily practice over many years. Take the time in treatment necessary to become a master at living your life.

23. After you are off painkillers, treatment focuses on staying sober, rebuilding your life, healing, and realizing joy.

You know you are in recovery when you are not hurting yourself through addicting and are living a productive, meaningful, and joyful life.

I will talk about renouncing addicting in a later lesson. Suffice it to say for now that you are better off if you stop harming yourself in any way by addicting. If you stop addicting, you will be in a better position to repair and heal your life.

Let's talk now about healing and repair. You will need to heal from any psychiatric or medical illnesses you have. You may have to heal from the trauma of abuse and neglect. You will also have to heal from the traumas that your addiction brought.

You will also need to repair your life. You may have to rehabilitate both your career and your relationships. Be patient and persistent. Seek treatment to rebuild and repair yourself and your life.

Finally, work with your therapist to realize a fulfilling, joyful life. When you are leading a joyful, fulfilling, meaningful, loving, and harmonious life, you will likely feel so good that life will be too good to throw away for the temporary high of a painkiller. Make sure you devote yourself to a daily spiritual practice and involve yourself in some sort of spiritual community to cultivate your spirituality.

When you are living mindfully, with a humble and reverent appreciation for this gift of consciousness—for this sacred moment—your relationship to distress will change. You will not feel so hooked by painful experience. Your practice of mindful appreciation will take the suffering out of distress. You will feel free, and will develop the capacity to experience peace amid the storm. Your practice of mindful appreciation will promote your resilience in the face of adversity. It will protect you from readdicting.

You will realize joy when you devote yourself to nurturing and savoring Life. Live for something greater than yourself. Live for a larger purpose than mere gratification or relief-seeking. Look and listen inwardly to the stirrings of your soul. What are you called to do? What does love ask of you? Devote yourself to a life of love—to taking the High Road—and you will ultimately experience such peace, mental calmness, and joy that you never need to addict again.

PART III
What You Need to Know
about Getting Sober

24. You can be addiction-free.

At times, you have probably have felt hopeless about your addiction. You may feel your addiction is so strong that you are helpless to overcome it. You may also feel that there is no way out, that you have no options. You may feel that your situation is unique. You may think that others may be able to overcome their painkiller addiction, but that you are not like others.

If you feel lost in the darkness of your addiction, take heart. Everyone who has overcome their painkiller addiction has felt just as you do. And no matter how bleak or desperate your situation, no matter how severe your addiction, know that there is someone out there who has felt just like you, but who has become addiction-free. You, too, can be addiction-free, just like the roughly thirty million people in the United States who have gone into remission from their addiction.

All it takes is good treatment and a willingness on your part to do the work of recovery. No one recovers alone, so you will also need to become humble and allow others to help and support you. Treatment works, if you are willing to do the work required of you and you get the treatment you need.

There are many paths to recovery, and each person's healing journey is unique. Because you are unique, you will need individualized treatment that addresses your unique needs and preferences. Find treatment providers who seek to understand you, explain to you your many treatment options, and provide the treatment that respectfully meets your needs and preferences.

A lot of people are dying from this disease. But, you don't have to die. You don't have to go to an institution...jail. You can be successful. It's a disease—not curable, but it's manageable.

Daniel, 38

We live in a very hopeful time for people who are caught in the addiction trap. For example, extremely effective medication treatments for opioid use disorder (painkiller addiction) exist. Each medication has its pros and cons, but these medications are saving millions of lives. The odds are that one of these medications will also help you.

Good addiction treatment is also becoming more available. Many addiction treatment providers can see you remotely with video conferencing if access to care is a problem. You might find you prefer videotherapy for therapy sessions because it is so convenient. If you do videotherapy, make sure you're working with a licensed and credentialed therapist. Your therapist will either use a confidential and secure videoconferencing platform, or will ask you to sign your permission to use a non-secure platform such as Skype or FaceTime. Your therapist will also likely ask you for a copy of your ID to prove your identity and may ask for proof of residence. Your therapist needs to know where you physically are at the times of your sessions in case there is an emergency.

New web-based technology applications have also become available to support your recovery. These applications can help promote your sobriety by providing coaching, motivation, and encouragement. A few options include:

- CBT4CBT (www.cbt4cbt.com)
- reSET-O (https://peartherapeutics.com/products/reset-reset-o/)
- WeConnnect (https://www.weconnectrecovery.com)
- I Am Sober (www.iamsober.com)

You will need support in your recovery. You can develop good recovery supports from one of the many mutual help groups available to you, such as Narcotics Anonymous. Whatever your preference might be, know that there is a recovery support group out there for you.

After you become sober, you will need to address the pain that drove you to addiction in the first place. If you have other psychiatric illnesses or medical illnesses, you will need treatment for these. You may have a history of trauma or neglect. If so, you will need treatment to heal your emotional brain and develop the capacity to love and be loved in healthy ways.

25. You can turn your addiction into a blessing.

Right now you may be suffering terribly, so what I'm about to say may sound strange. But if you deal with your addiction properly, your addiction may be the best thing that ever happened to you! Your addiction could be the best gift of all. It is true. Just ask one of the millions of people in recovery who went into the furnace of addiction and came out a star. Their addiction turned them into beautiful people living beautiful lives.

Why is this? The reason is because their addiction forced them to grow psychologically and spiritually in order to survive. Mediocrity was not an option anymore.

Many people are driven by their needs for safety, comfort, and connection. Fear and greed govern their actions. The ego is in charge, rather the Higher Self, or the force of love.

If you look closely and honestly at your life, you will see that it was your need for comfort that drew you into the abyss of addiction, not love. But it is love that will get you out.

Your addiction has likely visited upon you much suffering, defeat, loss, shame, humiliation, and despair. You have struggled. You have known tremendous pain. It is this pain that now forces you to grow and transform.

Through your recovery, you will develop the capacity to live out of love rather than out of fear and greed. Recovery requires that you love yourself and others, so you will only act in ways that enhance Life.

Your suffering will give you a deeper appreciation for Life. You will develop compassion not only for yourself, but for our fellow humans who also suffer as you have. You will develop a gentle, forgiving, and understanding nature. You will develop wisdom. You will learn how to live life skillfully so as to minimize your pain and any pain you might inflict upon others. You will develop virtue.

The thing I would say to others is don't wait so long to get sober. Don't be embarrassed. Get help. You're not going get better hiding your problem.

David, 43

You will also learn to accept the many pains that life visits upon you. You will learn to not make an enemy out of distress. When you do this, your suffering will leave you. You will be free. Perhaps for the first time, you will experience peace, even during difficult times.

Through your recovery, you will develop the capacity to share yourself with others and allow them to help you. By cultivating your humility and integrity, you will earn the privilege of loving connections with others. Through your practice of love, you will become a member of a loving community that will support and sustain you through difficult times.

You will also experience the greatest gift of all—the gift of giving. You will live to nurture both your life and the lives of all those you touch. This will give you a sense of meaning that is far greater than a sense of gratification.

As humans, it is our privilege not only to live life out of love and thus to nurture life, but to also consciously savor Life. Through your spiritual practice, you will develop the capacity to experience the joy of simply being alive. You will experience the extraordinary in the ordinary, and the miraculous in the mundane. Through the practice of presence, this moment just as it is will be more than enough. Any urges to addict to realize "something more" will evaporate.

Your pain is a gift. It will force you to grow and find another way to realize authentic joy. That way is recovery. By doing your recovery work, you will transform the curse of your addiction into the greatest blessing of your life.

26. There are many paths to living addiction-free.

In another book I wrote, *The Joy of Recovery: A Path to Freedom from Addiction,* I discuss the following twelve universal touchstones of recovery that you must address in order to lead a stable, joyful, and addiction-free life.

1. Work on recovery.
2. Create a positive recovery environment.
3. Renounce addicting.
4. Act with integrity.
5. Heal.
6. Love.
7. Respect reality.
8. Grow.
9. Persevere.
10. Develop healthy relationships.
11. Take accountability.
12. Cultivate your spirituality.

You must do the work of these touchstones to recover from your addiction, but how you do this work is up to you. There is no one right way.

Emotional support is essential to your recovery. You have many options for recruiting recovery supports from many different types of mutual help meetings.

You will benefit from a recovery mentor or coach with whom you can check in. Recovery mentors and coaches provide essential one-on-one supervision, accountability, support, and guidance. Again, you have many options. You could obtain a sponsor or a mentor from one of the other mutual help meetings. You could also hire a professional recovery coach.

You might benefit from individual and/or group therapy, especially if you also have another psychiatric illness or are a survivor of trauma or neglect.

If you like the twelve-step support groups, then working on the steps with a sponsor can be life-changing. The twelve steps have proven to be extremely effective for healing, growth, and transformation.

You will want to engage in some sort of daily spiritual practice. Spend a part of every day in silence and stillness. This will give you the clarity and perspective you need to navigate life peacefully and wisely. Again, you have many options. These include prayer, meditation, yoga, and contemplation.

Consider journaling. Journaling brings to the surface what lies just below your awareness. Journaling promotes clarity. Journaling is a great way to tap the reservoir of wisdom that lies within you.

There are many books, videos, and podcasts on recovery. You might want to set a goal for yourself to read at least ten pages a day or listen to a thirty-minute podcast. Read or listen to absorb the wisdom so that your reading and listening transform you.

Whatever you decide to do, do it! Don't wait for someone to fix you. Recovery only benefits those who do the work. Make sure you think, talk, read, or write about recovery every day. Create daily and weekly schedules of recovery activities and rituals. Make recovery your first priority and don't let life get in the way. Remember, without your recovery you have nothing else.

27. Renounce all addicting at once rather than one addiction at a time.

Cross-addiction is common, meaning that you may stop painkillers but continue addicting in other ways, such as smoking. To be in true recovery, you want to renounce all addicting out of your new commitment to managing pain, urges, and impulses in loving ways that don't harm you or anyone else.

Renunciation gets a bad rap. You may think of it as deprivation. This could not be further from the truth. Instead, when you renounce addicting, several good things happen:

- *You feel a renewed sense of safety.* It becomes clear to you that addicting is harmful and that it is best for you not to addict. There are no gray zones. You must simply abstain from addicting.

- *You notice your cravings subside, because addicting to one substance or behavior triggers cravings for your other addictions.* You strengthen your recovery.

- *Living requires less work* because you don't have to invest effort into attempting to manage cravings, compulsions, and the negative consequences of addicting. You are less distracted, more focused, and more productive.

- *Life becomes much more satisfying, as you experience true freedom and lack of impairment.* Guilt fades as life becomes more coherent. You can bask in the satisfying feeling of doing the right thing. You are living according to your conscience when you don't hurt yourself by addicting.

- *Self-efficacy grows, meaning that you have control over your actions and your life.* You feel more empowered. With empowerment you become more accountable for your life. Your accountability then enhances your success.

- *With no addictive outlet for managing stress and pain, you are forced to cope with life on life's terms.* Creativity and problem solving improve. You learn to resolve emotional pain with love rather than numb it with pleasure.

- *You stop hurting yourself.* This adds to the quality, vitality, and length of your life.

I encourage you to renounce all addicting as a supreme act of self-love. In recovery, you take on the responsibility of taking care of yourself as if you were your own beloved child. Out of reverence for yourself, you would do nothing to harm yourself, including addicting. Right? With the gift of this one precious life we are also given the responsibility for caring for our life. Since addicting is self-destructive, it is simply something that we should not do.

How do you develop your capacity for renunciation? Follow these steps:

- *Know that it is easier to give up all addictions at once rather than one at a time.* Ask yourself if you would rather go through one period of withdrawal or several episodes of withdrawal. If you are in rehab, it is far easier to give up everything at once while you are in a "time-out" from the stresses of your everyday life.

- *Know that if you renounce all addicting, you will increase your chance of recovery from painkillers by about 25 percent.* This is likely due to the fact that you are not going through the stressful stimulation and withdrawal of addicting anymore.

- *Cultivate your reverence for Life.* To renounce addicting is to perform an act of worship to Life. It is a formal dedication to a no-harm way of being, seeing, and doing. Take responsibility for taking very good care of yourself.

- *Have courage to deal with your distress. Manage your pain with love for yourself.* Ask for help.

- *Practice the craving management techniques that I talk about in a later lesson for all of your addictions.*

Recovery is a way of being, seeing, and doing in which you eventually realize joy, fulfillment, and meaning. By renouncing all addicting, you take the first crucial step toward realizing the full fruits of recovery.

28. Learn to moderate rewards.

Because you suffer from addiction, you need to moderate rewards. What does this mean?

Addiction has damaged your brain's drive-reward system. When you took painkillers, your brain really liked them. The opioids intensely stimulated the pleasure-reward system of your brain. Your brain responded to this intense reward by creating intense cravings for more. You know what this has been like for you. Your cravings led to strong urges to use more painkillers, and you lost control. That's when your addiction set in.

You likely have a genetic vulnerability to addiction. Some people just don't get that much pleasure out of painkillers. Or, if they do feel good, they still don't have a desire for more after they wear off. That probably wasn't the case for you.

As I talked about in the previous lesson, cross-addiction is common. This means that if you have one addiction, such as to painkillers, you are vulnerable to having more than one addiction, such as alcohol.

Because of this, you will need to be careful when it comes to hedonic substances and behaviors. "Hedonic" means pleasure-inducing. These include addictive substances such as alcohol, cocaine, methamphetamine, cannabis, sugar, and nicotine. It also includes pleasurable activities such as sex, spending, and gambling. One or more of these hedonic substances or behaviors may be a risk for you.

Take an honest look at yourself. What other addictive substances or activities induce intense pleasure (reward) and also lead to strong cravings for more? You want to be careful with these substances and behaviors. Remember that you have a vulnerable drive-reward system.

Regarding addictive behaviors and food, we cannot completely renounce eating, sex, using the Internet, or spending. With these, we need to be very mindful. I find the most important question is whether we are engaging in these behaviors to soothe ourselves or out of a sense that we lack something. The trick here is to do three things: One, commit to managing any distress you might have in non-addictive ways. Two, devote yourself to doing other non-addictive things that are fun and rewarding. Three, cultivate your spirituality, including the practice of presence, so that this moment is more than enough, just as it is. If you are living a joyful life, you won't feel an emptiness that you need to addict to fill.

For example, if you eat compulsively to soothe yourself, you need to learn to eat mindfully primarily for fuel, rather than for pleasure. Eating then becomes an intentional practice. It is purpose over pleasure. When it comes to eating, this means the purpose of eating to sustain your health and vitality is more important than the pleasure of eating. Pleasure is nature's way of motivating us to do things that are good for us. If we live just for pleasure, however, we risk losing sight of what is good for us.

Recovery requires a change of attitude. You need to now devote yourself to feeling good by doing things that are fulfilling and meaningful, rather than things that are intensely pleasurable. Pleasure is wonderful, but for you, too much pleasure can be too much of a good thing. It can be dangerous because it can damage your brain's drive-reward system and trigger addiction.

If you think about it, we're all in the same boat. Most of us feel the lure of seeking happiness through pleasure rather than seeking fulfillment through meaning. Whether we are in recovery or not, part of our spiritual growth includes an elevation of our life agenda. When we die, what will matter most is not how much we stimulated our brain's drive-reward system. Sensual pleasures are wonderful, but they do not make for a meaningful life. What matters most is that we lead loving, meaningful lives, living true to the deepest callings of our Higher Selves.

Let this be your new life agenda. Be cautious of intensely pleasurable substances and activities. Make the moderation of rewards part of your daily self-care.

29. Although you might feel emotional distress, you don't have to suffer.

In life, distress is inevitable, but suffering is optional. You might be asking, "How can that be?" The answer is that mindfulness can take the suffering out of distress.

When you practice mindfulness, you do two things. First, you pay close attention to this present moment. You ask, "What is happening in this moment, right now?" You notice what you are feeling, hearing, seeing, and even thinking. You become present. In presence, you see that you are actually the still, empty Awareness that is experiencing what is arising. This separates you from your experience. You see you are not your experience. You don't have to take your experience, including whatever thoughts you may be having, personally. By paying attention to your experience, you develop the capacity for freedom. With practice, you will develop the freedom to act or not act according to what is best for you, regardless of your urges to do otherwise.

The second thing you do in mindfulness is accept what you are experiencing without judgment. This is a practice of an attitude of unconditional acceptance of all experience. With practice—and it does take practice—you will eventually be able to experience pain with acceptance. With acceptance, there is distress, but suffering goes away.

Mindful acceptance of your experience brings about compassion. Let's say you find yourself experiencing shame, self-hatred, anger, or painful traumatic memories. Your usual response may be to numb your pain in any way you can. Instead, be with your pain with an attitude of appreciation. What then naturally arises is the experience of loving self-compassion for your pain. Your self-compassion eases your suffering.

What made me finally wake up was realization that I'd had enough pain. Enough depression. Enough self-will. Enough lying and manipulating everyone and everything. I got tired of it. I was willing to listen to a therapist.

Ann, 47

Nonjudgmental acceptance of this moment exactly as it is is a spiritual practice. The idea is that we humbly embrace all experience, whether painful or pleasurable, with acceptance. We practice saying "thank you" for our experience, even when it is very painful. Our practice is to have an unconditional reverence for Reality. When we humbly and reverently say "yes" to what is, suffering diminishes.

Acceptance does not come naturally. Our nature is to judge pain and distress as negative, to run from it, to push it away, or to do something to get rid of it. That is why when you feel the distress of cravings or withdrawal, for example, there is an urge to take painkillers to take the pain away. It takes purposeful, repetitive practice to attend to our experience with an attitude of reverent acceptance.

Try it. If you respond with acceptance of the experiences of cravings and withdrawal, you will see that instead of addicting to numb the pain, you will be able to tolerate your distress. You will notice that compassion for your distress arises. Suffering diminishes as you develop the capacity to simply be with your experience.

Then, with the space and freedom mindfulness provides, you will notice you can reflect on what you can do to ease your distress. Perhaps you will ask someone for support. Or, maybe you will go for a walk in nature, listen to some good music, exercise, or take a bath. Mindfulness enables you to lovingly hold yourself in your pain and then do something to help you ease or bear your distress.

With your suffering diminished and your freedom enhanced, you don't have to impulsively or compulsively addict anymore to numb your pain. This mindfulness practice gives you the ability to love. And with love comes joy, even in the midst of distress.

Do this experiment and see for yourself. For the next ninety days, practice mindfully attending with acceptance and appreciation whenever distress arises. In ninety days, see if your suffering has diminished. You will discover for yourself that while distress is inevitable, suffering is optional.

30. You will need a supportive environment to get sober.

Recovery requires a supportive environment. Without the proper environment, you are doomed to fail. Create an "8-S" environment as the foundation for your recovery. An 8-S environment is one that is safe, supportive, stable, sober, low stress, structured, supervised, and has therapeutic sequellae ("sequellae" are things that happen as a result of your behavior). Let's take a close look at each of these eight requirements.

Safety is the first order of business in your recovery. Remove any immediate or potential threats to your safety. Once you feel safe, you can work on your recovery.

Supportive: We need each other to get by. Just as someone might need a cane to stay upright, so you need the emotional support of others to stay in remission. No one does recovery alone.

Surround yourself with healthy people who care about you. Let yourself be held accountable. You need mirrors in your life to reflect to you both the positive and the negative so you can feel good about the positive and correct the negative. Humbly let others mentor and guide you through your healing and recovery.

You will need a recovery mentor and other recovery supports. Use them to talk out cravings and to get support and guidance based on their recovery experience.

Stable: Recovery requires stability, as instability can lead to a recurrence of addicting. You need a stable living situation and work environment. You need stable relationships, especially with your recovery supports. You need stable life routines. You can't work on your recovery with your life up in the air.

Sober: If you don't want to slip, stay away from the slippery places. Don't expose yourself to people or places where painkillers are available to you.

It's difficult to end sometimes-lifelong relationships with others who suffer from addiction. But this is something you must do to create a sober environment for yourself. Also, don't associate with those with less than a few years of recovery. Their fragility can trigger re-addicting. Cravings can be infectious.

Low stress: One of the most common causes of addicting is stress. Minimize your stress to protect your recovery. Live a simple, balanced, and routine life.

Structured: We drift without structured, daily routines. Positive routines promote recovery. Examples include a structured recovery program, an exercise program, time with friends and family, and time for your spiritual practice.

Structure includes not only your daily commitments to yourself, but also your daily external commitments to others, such as to work, child care, volunteer work, and school. Having these external structures protects you from boredom and keeps you engaged with life.

Supervised: The mind can be a dangerous place; don't go in there alone. Share your thoughts, feelings, and actions with others. This includes your recovery mentor, recovery supports, friends, and family members. Allow these people to supervise you. This provides support and creates accountability.

Allowing yourself to be supervised requires humility. It requires acknowledging you have an illness that can kill you and that you need help. Allow yourself to become humble.

Supervision gives you feedback and direction about your recovery work, your psychological status, your spiritual status, and your relationship status. Coaching in these areas helps you progress in your recovery.

Therapeutic sequellae: The consequences, or things that happen as a result of your behavior. This includes positive consequences of positive actions and negative consequences of unskillful actions. Your recovery environment should include both positive and negative consequences that result in personal growth.

Have the courage to put yourself in an accountable environment where good things happen when you do good things and you experience the natural painful consequences of addicting or otherwise behaving destructively. Don't allow others to enable you, no matter how great the temptation. Painful consequences force you to learn, grow, and change for the better.

What I learned most in recovery is how to love myself again and accept the person that I am. I've also learned that recovery is not a race to the finish. For me, the process has taken several years. Each step of the way I've learned something new.

Jack, 45

Your environment is of supreme importance. Create a solid foundation for your recovery by creating a supportive recovery environment. Humbly ask for help—you cannot be your only support.

31. Never allow yourself to hurt alone.

Pain fuels addiction. If you're like most people, you used painkillers to numb both physical and emotional pain. Isolation also fuels addiction. Pain plus isolation leads to addiction. You may have fallen into addiction because when you were hurting, you were also disconnected from others. When you are hurting alone, addicting to numb your pain can be irresistible.

You can protect yourself from addicting by making a rule for yourself that you will never hurt alone. Some say the opposite of addiction is connection. If you are connected to others, you can let others help you when you are in pain. Remember that a pain shared is a pain halved.

We need each other to get by. Life is difficult. It is often painful. We simply cannot endure and resolve all our problems on our own. Even if we could, it is incredibly lonely and painful to live this way. Life is a team sport. Just as others need you, you also need others.

When you grew up, did you feel connected to people who loved you? Were your caregivers tuned into you? Did they know when you were hurting? Did they intervene to guide, reassure, and support you through your pain? If you had this loving connection growing up, then you are fortunate.

If you did not have this kind of emotional support growing up, then you are a survivor of emotional neglect. You probably grew up feeling emotionally alone. You also hurt alone, and have continued to hurt alone to this day. You lost the instinct to turn to others for help, because there was no one there to help when you were hurting. You parents may have been well meaning, but they may have been busy dealing with the hardships of their own lives, or they may have been emotionally disabled themselves, not knowing how to tune in and connect with you in order to be there for you. They may have been emotionally neglected themselves when they were growing up. The trauma of emotional neglect can get passed on from generation to generation.

If you are a neglect survivor, then hurting alone feels natural. Addicting to numb your pain probably then feels just as natural, as this may seem like the only option you have. At this point in life, sharing your pain with others may seem as unnatural as jumping off a cliff and just as scary. If others were never there for you before, how could it possibly be that they could be there for you now?

This is where your intentions come in. You have to do what you know is good for you even if it feels uncomfortable and scary. Look at it this way: You have an emotional disability, and you need emotional rehabilitation, just like someone else might need physical rehabilitation for a physical disability.

Make a commitment to connect on a daily basis. Commit to "get current" with at least one person every day before you go to bed. "Getting current" means telling someone safe and trustworthy everything that has happened and everything you are thinking, feeling, and doing. Do this with friends, family, a recovery mentor, or a recovery support, especially if you are having cravings.

Make getting current a daily recovery practice. While it may be awkward at first, with practice it will eventually become second nature. Your connection will protect you from addiction.

You are not meant to live life alone. Protect yourself from the pain and isolation that fuel addiction by living by the rule, "Never hurt alone."

32. Never crave alone.

The first rule of craving management is to never crave alone. The first instant you get a thought of taking a painkiller, tell someone. Pick up the phone and talk to your recovery mentor or other recovery supports. Do this each and every time you get a thought of addicting, even if it is a hundred times a day!

Asking for help requires mindfully taking a step back from your cravings when they first arise. Realize that you are in trouble. See how you experience the state of mind in which you say, "To hell with it." In these times, you don't care about the consequences of addicting and just want a painkiller. Note the feeling of not caring about yourself or anyone else. See how you feel that nothing and no one can stop you from addicting. When you observe yourself having his attitude, separate yourself from the attitude by mindfully noting it and ask for help immediately.

Talk out your cravings. When you talk to someone about your cravings you want to talk about four things:

- The good things that will happen if you don't addict

- The bad things that will likely happen if you addict

- What triggered the craving? Cravings usually arise when we are distressed. They are a signal that your well-being is compromised. How are you not right with Life? Are you stressed, bored, upset? What is blocking your experience of joy and abundance?

- What can you do to resolve the roots of cravings? Remember that recovery involves managing emotional pain with love. What can you do to nurture and soothe yourself? What can you do to cultivate feelings of joy and abundance?

Make a "consequences card" to carry with you at all times in your wallet or purse. On one side, put all the good things that will come with recovery. On the other side, put all the bad things that will happen if you addict. Think about biological, psychological, social, and spiritual consequences. Update your consequences card as you think of new things. At some point, go to an office supply store to laminate your consequences card so that it will not fall apart with use. Every time you talk out your cravings, refer to your consequences card.

Talking out your cravings does two important things. First, it strengthens connections between the part of your brain that knows what is best for you and your brain's disordered drive-reward system. Every time you talk out cravings, you change your brain, enhancing your ability to do what is right regardless of cravings to do otherwise.

The second benefit of talking out cravings is that it connects you to people who care about you so that you can get help to resolve your distress. To ask for help, you have to have a healthy network of recovery supports—people who can help you manage your cravings. One of the first tasks of recovery is to develop this support network. Most people develop recovery supports by going to mutual help meetings such as SMART Recovery, Refuge Recovery, or Narcotics Anonymous. (See lesson 66 on support group meetings.)

Practice "Never crave alone" over and over, until you become adept at it. Talking out cravings and other recovery practices are just like any other skill. You learn craving management skills by practicing them over and over. With practice you, too, will learn how to manage your cravings!

33. There are many ways to manage cravings.

In addition to the rule, "Never crave alone," you have many other ways to manage cravings. There may be times when you cannot reach someone to talk out your cravings. Carry a journal with you so that you can express your swirl of emotions in writing; this may help you work through your cravings on your own if no other support is available. When cravings arise, practice the following "Four-Rs" technique to work through cravings:

1. *Recognize* when you are having cravings. Notice the very first thought of addicting. Get very present. Be the Awareness that is experiencing the craving, so that you don't get lost in the craving.

2. *Resist* acting on the craving. Write in your journal about the good things that follow recovery and the bad things that follow addicting.

3. *Relax* into your cravings. Don't fight them or make them an enemy. Instead, welcome them as a signal that you are not right with Life. Listen to your cravings. What is triggering them? You may want to write in your journal about what pain might be triggering your cravings. Write about what pain is blocking your experience of joy.

4. *Return* to a state of mindful presence. Now do "the next right thing." Do one of a thousand things to soothe and care for yourself. This will help distract you from your cravings. In time, they will go away—they always do. As you continue to nurture yourself, you will gradually transform your cravings into joy.

Practice these Four Rs with patience, perseverance, and faith. With practice, your brain will slowly change, and you will develop freedom from your cravings.

There are other ways to manage cravings. Pick a few of these to practice on a daily and weekly basis:

- *"Make friends" with your cravings.* Don't make them an enemy. Remember that attitude is everything. Practice an attitude of reverent acceptance of cravings. Smiling at your cravings takes the suffering out of distress. Comfort yourself with the reminder that all experience, including cravings, comes and goes.

- *Make a gratitude list.* Carry it in your wallet or purse. When you get a craving, pull out your gratitude list and reflect on all your blessings and what you will lose if you act on your cravings.

- *Go to in-person recovery meetings.* Seek out the fellowship of others who are practicing recovery. If an in-person meeting is not immediately available, you can always attend an online meeting, such as those at (www.smartrecovery.org) or (www.intherooms.com).

- *See a therapist once or twice a week.* Or, attend a substance abuse treatment group. You will benefit from therapy to manage pain and live more skillfully, especially in the first one to five years of early recovery.

- *Exercise.* Exercise is a great way to work off stress and get your endorphins flowing.

- *Pray or meditate twice a day or more.* The refuge of stillness is always available to you when you are distressed to keep you from getting swept away by your cravings.

- *Attend religious/spiritual/inspirational meetings.* The stimulation and support of these meetings will enhance and sustain your vitality.

- *Practice yoga, tai chi, or qigong.* These mind-body practices soothe and cultivate the experience of stillness in motion. They will help to ground you and soothe you.

- *Go for long walks.* Expose yourself to the rejuvenating effects of being in nature.

- *Read spiritual/inspirational/recovery literature, watch recovery videos, or listen to podcasts on recovery.* Remember that you want to be thinking about, talking about, and practicing recovery every day as your first priority.

- *Engage in productive activities to distract yourself.* Ask yourself, "What is the best thing for me to do right now?" Substitute cravings with a feeling of accomplishment.

- *Volunteer.* The practice of service to others is profoundly fulfilling and goes a long way toward filling the emptiness that can drive cravings. Doing service to others is an effective way to "get outside of oneself."

- *Give to someone.* Call on a friend who's had a death in the family. Do an errand for someone in need of help. Practice generosity on a regular basis to cultivate happiness and joy.

- *Continue to meditatively sit with your cravings.* Practice "urge surfing"—watch your cravings like clouds in the sky of Awareness and wait for the cravings to pass. Intentionally and gently abstain from acting on the compulsions that arise. Instead, be still. Be the Awareness that you are, separate from urges to addict.

- *Envision the life you want to live.* Imagine how acting on your cravings will and will not help you achieve your life vision. Each day, visualize how you are going to practice nurturing and savoring Life.

- *Label cravings as just cravings and do not give yourself a choice.* Remind yourself that every time you do not act on a craving, you strengthen your recovery. Label the craving as a signal of distress and not acting on cravings as the "feeling of healing." Imagine how good you will feel when the craving has passed without addicting.

- *Distance yourself from any triggers.* Get out of any high-risk or dangerous situations. Stay away from high-risk people.

- *Continue to relax.* Use deep-breathing and muscle-relaxation techniques.

- *Mindfully note when rationalizations or justifications for addicting arise.* Go over your thinking with your recovery mentor, therapist, or a recovery support. Work to get clarity on your "mis-thinking."

- *Practice thought-stopping techniques.* Thought-stopping not only helps when you are having cravings, it also helps when you are beating yourself up or having other negative thoughts. Say "stop" out loud, visualize a stop sign, or snap a rubber band on your wrist. Note the thought and direct your attention back to the Present. Identify the next right thing to do. Then do it without hesitation. Substitute craving thoughts with positive thoughts and images, such as images of healing, your ideal self, a future goal, or images of loved ones. Pull out photographs of loved ones. You can also substitute craving thoughts with reflections on your consequences card. Reflect on the positive consequences of not addicting.

- *When cravings arise, don't "entertain the thought."* Don't romance the addiction, thinking about the pleasure of addicting. This only seduces you into obsessing over "temporary gain" without seeing the much greater "long-term pain." Remind yourself that addictive gratification is no substitute for the fulfillment of love.

- *Some people benefit from medications to reduce cravings.* For some, cravings are too powerful and craving management skills are too weak to manage cravings without medications. There is nothing wrong with using medication to help manage cravings as long as you do not use the medication as a substitute for recovery work.

- *Address your pain with problem solving, perspective taking, or acceptance.* If the problem, for example, is that you are lonely, pick up the phone or go to a meeting rather than numbing loneliness by addicting.

- *Soothe yourself.* Treat yourself to something pleasurable that will not harm you or others. It might be a snack, entertainment, reading a good book, exercising, taking a bath, or playing a game.

- *Distract yourself by playing and having fun.* Busy yourself with reading, doing puzzles, knitting, playing a musical instrument, making models, learning to do something new, taking a course, playing video games (assuming you do not have a tech addiction), going for a walk, listening to music, going to a movie, going dancing, going bowling, going to a sport event, making love, or doing research for a future project or event such as a vacation.

Remember that the key to a long and successful life of recovery is skillful management of emotional pain. Cravings are the first and foremost form of pain that you will need to master to succeed. Have faith! Like many others before you, you, too, can master your cravings by patiently and persistently practicing these techniques. As you do so, don't be afraid of failure. Failure is actually success in disguise, because we learn the most from our mistakes. Just get up each time you fall and keep trying.

34. You will need to manage internal triggers that prompt you to reach for a painkiller.
As mentioned earlier, triggers of cravings can be both external and internal. Internal triggers include negative emotional states (negativity) such as worry, anger, fear, hopelessness, loneliness, self-pity, self-hatred, envy, or boredom.

Most people focus more on the negative than the positive, creating "dis-ease" and thus the conditions for a recurrence of addicting. Identify negativity when it arises and do something positive about it. Techniques to counter negativity include:

1. *Label* thoughts and feelings as just thoughts and feelings you are having. Recognize a negative attitude for what it is—something you can change. Remind yourself that you are not your negative emotional states.

2. *Say "thank you"* to the thought or feeling, asking yourself what purpose it might serve you. Let them teach you. How are you not right with Reality? What do you need to be doing differently? Practice unconditional friendliness toward all internal experiences. Don't hold onto them, however. Let them pass.

3. *Inquire and correct.* Inquire into the roots of negative thoughts, asking if they are realistic or productive. Counter negative thoughts with reality-based thoughts. If someone criticizes you, for example, put whatever truth there might be into a balanced perspective where you appreciate yourself and accept your faults. If self-hatred arises, remind yourself of your immeasurable value despite your imperfections. If you experience nonacceptance of some person or situation, accept the person exactly as they are or the situation just as it is.

4. *Practice gratitude.* Make a gratitude list. Add to it as you think of new things to be grateful for. Intentionally focus on what is good in your life rather than what is bad.

5. *Talk it out.* Call someone or talk to someone in person. Talk out your feelings. Remember the rule, "Never hurt alone." In doing so, explore how your negativity affects you and shift your attitude to a more balanced, positive perspective. Try to identify any distortions, such as black-and-white thinking, seeing only the negative in a situation, or taking something personally that is not about you.

6. *Act.* Engage in positive, self-soothing, and fun activities. Take good care of yourself. Play. Connect with others for guidance, reassurance, and support. Help someone. If you are bored, do something you enjoy. If you are lonely, pick up the phone and call someone. Reach out. Get something done that will leave you feeling good.

7. *Regroup and recharge.* Most negativity is rooted in fear and hopelessness. Get affirmation from affirming people. Reflect on past accomplishments. Notice that even the most "hopeless" people have succeeded in recovery through faithful persistence. Read inspiring spiritual or recovery literature. Remind yourself that failure gives the opportunity to learn and grow. Practice realistic positivity.

The internal trigger boredom can trigger addicting. Here, the external trigger is a lack of stimulation. You can manage boredom in two ways. The first is to practice presence. If you pay close attention to this moment, you will experience the extraordinary nature of the ordinary, and boredom will dissolve. The second thing you can do for boredom is to engage in a pleasurable or meaningful activity. One practice is to think about all the people in your life that you care about, and then reach out to one or more of them.

The key to avoiding internal triggers boils down to living a joyful life. We will talk more about cultivating joy in a later lesson. If you are full of joy, then you will not experience internal triggers, and cravings will likely not arise. If they do, they will not bother you as much.

Most importantly, remember to practice an attitude of unconditional appreciation of your experience, even when negative emotional states arise. They are just a sign that you are in pain, and that you are somehow not right with Reality. Smile at your internal triggers. Let them teach you how to live life more skillfully.

35. You will also need to manage external triggers.

As mentioned earlier, external triggers are people, places, things, and situations that awaken cravings. Common external triggers include drugs, drug paraphernalia, bars, people using, drug dealers, neighborhoods where you got your supply, and places where you addicted. Protect yourself from these triggers by removing these cues from your life and avoiding the places where you addicted in the past.

People can be triggers. One common trigger is a call from a dealer. Dealers are predators. Their calls are tests to see if you are vulnerable to addicting. Calls from addicting "friends" can also trigger cravings.

Minimize people triggers as much as possible. One common practice is to change your cell phone number, e-mail, and social media sites to make it more difficult for negative influences to contact you.

Isolation is another external trigger caused by a lack of connection to others. It is said that "isolation is the Devil's workshop." The opposite of addiction is connection. Although it is good to spend some time each day in solitude, you want to be alone in the context of a network of healthy, loving connections to people who know what's going on with you and who care about you. Avoid isolation by connecting every day with someone. Practice getting current with at least one person every day. This will protect you from isolation.

Also, untreated psychiatric and medical illnesses can also be triggers. Minimize these triggers by getting professional help. Conflict, stress, and loss are all potential triggers, because these emotions trigger the impulse to numb pain by addicting. When pain arises, practice attending with appreciation while doing what you can to soothe yourself and get support.

Jobs that expose you to the object of your addiction can be triggers. If you work in an environment where drugs are used, your chances of recovery fall close to zero. As part of setting up a supportive recovery environment, you will likely have to change jobs.

The important thing is don't lose hope and don't dwell on the bad things that you did. Admit them and move on. The people who really love you will let you do that.

John, 36

The numbers and types of triggers are many. Although you must work to remove triggers from your life, you cannot protect yourself from all possible people, places, things, and situations. Stress, for example, is unavoidable, no matter how skillful you become at minimizing and managing it. You will need to learn to manage unavoidable triggers.

The first step to managing external triggers is to mindfully note when you are triggered. Sometimes the trigger can induce a subtle passing negative thought that takes root and grows in your mind, such as self-pity or resentment. You cannot manage triggers if you do not know you are being triggered. Once you note the trigger, tell yourself that you are in trouble and act to protect your recovery.

The second step is to resolve the trigger or remove yourself from the trigger as fast as possible. If you are at a party or event, excuse yourself. If you see someone on the street who could be a trigger, walk the other way. If someone offers you a drug, say "no" and leave.

Whatever the trigger, call someone as soon as possible to talk out the craving. Remember to never crave alone. Exercise one or more of the many craving management techniques discussed in previous lessons.

Do what you need to do to minimize external triggers in your life. Then become skillful through practice at managing the triggers you cannot avoid. With time and practice, the inevitable triggers of life will eventually not threaten you. In the meantime, ask for help and get support to stay safe.

36. Warning! Losing your tolerance to narcotics can be deadly.

Ironically, one of the most dangerous times in your recovery from painkiller addiction can be after you stop using painkillers for a while. Why? Because you lose the tolerance that you had built up.

As you became addicted to painkillers, your brain "neuroadapted." In other words, your brain developed a tolerance, so that you needed more and more painkillers to get the same effect.

As you know, if you stop using painkillers, you will go through withdrawal. Withdrawal is the process of your brain getting used to not being on painkillers. Every day that you don't use painkillers, you lose your tolerance. Eventually your tolerance will diminish to where it was before you started using painkillers.

Ironically, rates of fatal overdoses are highest when you have just completed detox. We see this all the time in people discharged from detoxification treatment. If they were using a certain number of painkillers before they went into the hospital, and go home and use the same amount of pills again, the result can be death. This also happens to people who go through withdrawal in jail and then are released.

If you've been off painkillers for as little as a few weeks, you can lose the tolerance you once had for the drug. As a result, there is a chance that you could overdose despite your best intentions. Let's say you used to take ten Oxycontin tablets to get high. Then, you got off the drugs and are no longer using—your tolerance diminishes. What if you relapsed, and decided to take ten Oxycontins like you used to? With no tolerance built up, it could cause you to stop breathing and die.

Every year about 72,000 people in the United States die from drug overdoses. Many of them die due to drug use after they have lost their tolerance. If you have lost your tolerance, be extra careful if you find yourself slipping back into addiction. Know that the amount you safely took before could kill you now.

If you feel your addiction starting to flare up, ask for help right away before it is too late. You can best protect yourself by never hurting alone and by telling someone the very first moment the thought arises of using a painkiller. As long as you are connected to your recovery supports and are engaged in treatment, you will likely be able to nip readdiction in the bud.

37. You can manage physical pain without narcotics.

Do you have chronic physical pain? If so, you may feel that you've tried everything, and that narcotics are the only thing that works. You may also fear that your pain will be unbearable if you come off narcotics. You fear that not only will your pain increase, but you will also have the pain of withdrawal. Getting off narcotics may seem more difficult than taking a hike to the moon.

If you feel this way, and you now suffer from an addiction to narcotics, then you probably feel you are trapped in a cycle of despair. You can't live with painkillers, and you can't live without them.

Don't despair. There is good news! You can get off of narcotics and manage your pain without them. In fact, you'll find you feel much better than you do now with good non-narcotic management of your pain.

The first thing you should know is that narcotics often make pain worse. Pain actually gets better when you get off narcotics. Why is this? It is because narcotics lower your pain threshold. Your pain threshold is the amount of pain it takes to cause you distress. When you take narcotics long term, you become more sensitive to pain. You become less able to tolerate it. When you come off narcotics, your pain tolerance will go back up. As your pain threshold increases, your pain won't bother you as much.

The second thing you should know is that good pain treatment will allow you to live with your chronic pain without suffering. A recent study in the *Journal of the American Medical Association,* for example, showed that people with osteoarthritis treated with non-narcotic pain treatment did just as well as people treated with narcotics, but with fewer side effects.

The third thing you should know is that good pain management often involves a team of providers giving you several different treatments at once. This is called "multimodal pain management." You may receive different types of pain medications, such as acetaminophen and nonsteroidal anti-inflammatory agents (such as Motrin and Aleve). You may receive a medication to increase your pain threshold, such as duloxetine (brand name *Cymbalta*) or nortriptyline (brand name *Pamelor*). You may benefit from massage, acupuncture, yoga, or physical therapy.

Pain psychotherapy can help you to improve your functioning and to live comfortably with your pain. This therapy helps you to substitute negative and hopeless thoughts with more positive and realistic thoughts. It also empowers you to take charge of your life and not let pain take over. Your pain therapist will also help you to develop a practice of mindful acceptance to reduce your suffering.

With good treatment, you don't have to suffer any longer. You may not be completely pain-free, but you will be suffering-free.

Getting good non-narcotic pain treatment now will make it easier to get off your painkillers. If you can come off painkillers slowly over several months, you won't need treatment for withdrawal. If you need to get off painkillers quickly, combine good pain treatment with treatment for your withdrawal.

When you transition to non-narcotic, multimodal pain management, it may seem like things are getting worse before they get better. Take heart. This is normal. After a week or two, your physical pain will likely start to get better.

Talk to your doctor about multimodal, non-narcotic treatment for your pain. If he or she cannot provide this to you, ask for a referral to someone who can.

PART IV
What You Need to Know about Recovery

38. When it comes to recovery, you have choices.

Addiction is a disease of impaired choice. When you are caught up in the vortex of active addiction, you have impaired mind control and your ability to make good choices is diminished. You didn't choose to be this way, which is why addiction is not your fault.

Although you might choose when and where you use painkillers, your compulsions and cravings take away your choice to use or not to use. There is a loss of free will. Your addiction makes you feel at times as if someone else were controlling your actions. Your brain's drive-reward system has hijacked the part of your brain that makes reasonable decisions.

It is true that addiction impairs your capacity to choose— but only to a degree. Although you may feel you have no choice but to addict, this feeling is not the complete truth. The truth is that you do have choices, even when it feels that you do not. Most importantly, you have a choice to choose recovery. You can choose to ask for help. You can choose to get treatment. These choices are always available to you. Help is there. You need only to ask for it. You can choose to look around and see that recovery is a better way than addicting.

You have other choices as well. You can choose to learn to manage your pain without using painkillers. There are better ways. You can choose to bear your pain with the help and support of others while you figure out how to resolve pain through treatment and recovery work.

When you are addicted, your whole life agenda is devoted to trying to feel good and not feel bad by using painkillers. When you choose recovery, you have a choice to work on feeling good and not feeling bad through the practice of love. You can choose to work on feeling good through the fulfillment of loving yourself and others instead of through gratification.

What I've learned most in recovery is how to love myself again. I've also learned that recovery is not a race to the finish. For me, the process has taken several years. Each step of the way, I learn something new. You need to give 100 percent to your recovery. If you don't, it's not worth even trying to do it. You must be ready to be recovered.

Jack, 45

Hope is very powerful. You can choose to have hope by looking around you at all those who have successfully recovered from painkiller addiction and other illnesses and traumas. You can choose to have faith in the process of recovery, seeing that it works for even the most ill people who choose to do the work of recovery.

You can choose to work on your recovery every day. You can choose to open up and be authentic with safe people who want to support you in your recovery.

You can choose to act with integrity. You can choose to ask for help to do the next right thing, moment by moment. You can choose to be honest with yourself about the exact nature of things. You can choose to look Reality squarely in the eye. You can choose to be courageous.

You can choose to devote your life to something greater than yourself. You can live for a higher purpose that transcends your small personal concerns. You can choose to devote yourself to nurturing life in the ways that you are able.

You have a choice regarding your attitude. You can choose an attitude of appreciation for all that you have, even in your darkest times. You can always count your blessings, including the many people who are there to help you recover if you only choose recovery.

Rather than beating yourself up, wallowing in shame, and giving up, you can choose to forgive yourself, get up, and persist. You can look for the opportunities for learning, growth, and change in the midst of your difficulties.

You can choose to consider all that is happening in your life, whether painful or pleasurable, as teachers. You can choose to learn from painful experiences.

You can choose, right now, to committing to being your own ideal parent and treating yourself as your own cherished child. You can choose to be kind to yourself. You can choose to act in accordance with the fact that your life and all of life is of immeasurable worth. See that you have only this one precious life to live and then choose, with the help of others, to make your life the best life possible.

Although you didn't choose the cards you were dealt, you have a choice as to how to play them. You can choose to be a survivor rather than a victim. You can choose to work to make your trauma and misfortune sources of wisdom and growth rather than let them defeat you. You can choose to take accountability for your life, including accountability for asking for the help you need to succeed. In this way, you can choose to succeed.

You can choose humility. You can accept that you are broken, crooked, and flawed just like the rest of us. You can choose to be vulnerable with safe people who care about you.

You can choose to do what is good for you, even though it is unfamiliar and uncomfortable. You can choose to live life a better way than before, trying something new and good every day.

In the end, even though you suffer from an addiction that impairs your capacity to choose, you still have many choices. Most of all, choose to ask for help. Choose recovery.

39. Realize that life is sacred.

When I say that life is sacred, I mean that life—including your life—is of immeasurable value and is worthy of your utmost reverence. Think about that for a moment. Do you consider yourself to be worthy of utmost reverence? If you did consider yourself to be sacred, would you do anything to harm yourself? If you truly experienced the truth of your sacred nature, you would certainly get whatever help you needed to not addict. This is why reflecting on the sacred nature of existence will help you in your recovery.

A big part of spirituality involves opening our eyes to the basic truth of things—basic truths that we so easily forget even though they are right before our eyes. Spirituality involves countering our human habit of taking the miraculous for granted.

See the truth that you and all of life is sacred. Take note of the mystery of Awareness. How is it that the neural "symphony" of your brain creates the "music" of human awareness?

See that through the trillions of connections among the roughly eighty billion neurons that make up the cortex of your brain, you are the Universe aware of Itself. What this means is you are part of the Universe, and you are aware of the Universe, including yourself and others. See that you are part of a vast interconnected web of life that sustains you. See the astounding intelligence of nature that has brought you into existence. Nature has invested itself in you. You are one of nature's unique and astounding creations!

See also that you have but one brief moment of existence as a living human being on this planet before death. Like a flower, you bloom into the fullness of your life and then wilt and die. The fleeting, momentary nature of your existence gives a further sense of the preciousness of this one, unrepeatable, unique life that is yours.

Your life is precious beyond measure. You deserve to be treated—including by yourself—with the utmost reverence and respect. If you truly feel this fundamental truth to your core, you will never addict again.

Out of your seeing that this moment is sacred, commit yourself to the following recovery practices:

- *Kindness.* Treat both yourself and others with kindness.
- *Appreciation.* Appreciate yourself, others, and the gift of consciousness.
- *Care.* Care for yourself and others out of your reverence.
- *Respect.* Guard your own self-respect and treat others with respect.

- *Caution.* Be careful to not harm yourself or others or expose yourself or others to any unnecessary risks.
- *Generosity.* Seeing others as sacred, give of yourself to benefit others.
- *Tolerance and forgiveness.* Do not lose sight of the sacred nature of you and others in the face of hurtful behavior. Let go of judgment and condemnation, including judgments and condemnations of yourself. We are all imperfect. We all suffer. We all struggle with destructive impulses and lack of clarity at times. You didn't choose your genes or your parents. Neither did anyone else. See that everyone is just trying to get by as best they can, and that we all at times are deluded and unskilled.

Seeing that life is sacred inspires love. As you love the world, so the world loves you back. This love will fortify your recovery. You will want to do nothing to harm yourself or others. Your appreciation for this gift of existence dissolves the negativity that can lead to readdiction. It is all sacred, including hurt, anger, anxiety, grief, sadness, and other distressing emotions. The inevitable distresses of life are all but small waves on the still, deep ocean of your reverence, regardless of your conditions or circumstances.

40. A life of recovery is far better than a life of addicting.
You know full well that when you numb pain with painkillers, you multiply pain. You will never realize the joy you yearn for through your addiction. Ultimately, your addiction will ruin your life and may even kill you.

Yet you may not believe that recovery is a better way. Life without opioids may feel difficult, empty, dreary, boring, flat, or joyless. You may feel that the pain of life on life's terms is unbearable. You may feel that the pain of recovery is greater than the pain of addiction. If you feel this way, you probably have little hope that recovery offers a better way.

You are right that recovery can be painful, especially during the first year or two. You may suffer from PAWS. You may face trauma. Your addiction has likely visited upon you much wreckage and regret. It is true that life without opioids can be painful, especially at first.

However, I am here to tell you that facing and enduring your pain through recovery is a better way than trying to avoid your pain by numbing it in addiction. Emotional pain is not bad—it just hurts. That is okay. Pain never lasts forever. More importantly, your pain will transform you if you allow yourself to go through the process of legitimate suffering that is called "growth." Truly, pain is your friend. Facing and embracing your pain through recovery is the better way forward.

Through recovery you learn to endure and resolve your pain with love. You learn how to get by with the help of others. You learn to be accountable for your life. Recovery transforms you from victim to survivor. When you stop addicting, you can begin to heal. Recovery enables you to pull yourself together and repair your life.

Recovery also gives you the ability to start living a meaningful life. When you start to live for something greater than yourself, you will then begin to experience a quiet joy that is far better than the temporary opioid-induced roller coaster of euphoria and withdrawal. Recovery will rescue you from the prison of self-centered self-gratification. Recovery will give you the opportunity to realize your full, authentic self. It will give you the capacity to savor this gift of life unadulterated. It will give you the "something more" that you sought through painkillers.

If you give it time and do the work required of you, your recovery will deliver you from the torment of addiction. You must be patient, endure your pain with the support of others, and do the next right thing, moment by moment and day by day.

Have faith, knowing that everyone who does the work of recovery realizes the fruits of recovery. Look around you at the many people who were far worse off than you and who have realized joyful lives through their recovery. See that healing, growth, and transformation are possible for *anyone* who truly devotes themselves to their recovery.

A joyful and fulfilling life is awaiting you. All you need to do is to renounce addicting, ask for help, and live this day as best you can. If you take care of today, you will create a better tomorrow. Slowly, day by day, year by year, two steps forward and one step back, you will grow through the ups and downs

86

of recovery. While the death of your life of addiction can be painful, your rebirth in recovery will be well worth it.

41. You will need devotion to your well-being.

Recovery from addiction requires that you devote yourself to your well-being.

You may be thinking that you are devoted to your well-being. That's why you used painkillers, after all. They made you feel better. Right?

You would be right, except that painkillers make things worse in the long run. That's in part why they call it addiction. By using painkillers, you have inadvertently harmed your well-being.

It is true that you are devoted to feeling good and not feeling bad. But this is different from being devoted to your well-being. Sometimes what feels good is not good for us. That is the essence of addiction. When you are truly devoted to your well-being, you will do what is good for you, regardless of whether it feels good or not. You will not do anything that causes you harm, no matter how good it may feel in the moment. You will do what is right regardless of urges to do otherwise. This is why a devotion to your well-being is an act of integrity.

I continue to emphasize the point: You will need the help of others along the way. Remember that no one does recovery alone. You cannot take the best care of yourself without the help and guidance of others. We all need each other to get by. Don't live life alone. That is not what is best for you. Out of your devotion to your well-being, connect with healthy, loving people who can support you in your recovery.

Devotion to your well-being requires discipline. Being disciplined is actually a loving thing to do. Out of love for yourself, do what is good for you, even when it requires effort and you don't feel like it. Devotion to your well-being means you don't do what you necessarily feel like doing. You do what is best for you. You get up and exercise, for example, even if you feel like sleeping in. This is discipline. You eat one bite of pie rather than eating the whole piece. See that being disciplined is part of your devotion to your well-being.

Out of your devotion to your well-being, you commit to taking very good care of yourself. I discuss self-care in a later lesson.

Recovery is the practice of love: love for self, love for others, and love for life. Loving yourself by devoting yourself to taking good care of yourself is one aspect of the practice of love. If you are truly devoted to your well-being, you will do nothing to harm yourself, you will seek support when you are hurting, and you will ask for help when you experience cravings or other urges to act in ways that harm your well-being.

Knowing that you are sacred, devote yourself to your well-being. Be your own ideal parent. Nurture your well-being the way you would care for your own cherished child.

If you take good care of yourself, you will suffer less. If you suffer less, you will be less vulnerable to the urge to numb your pain through addicting. Commit to resolving your pain through loving self-care. Devote yourself from this day forward to your well-being. This is an essential part of your practice of recovery.

42. Recovery works if you do the work.

Recovery requires effort. Time and again, I see that my patients who do well are the ones who do the most work on their recovery. My patients who do not do well seem to hope that through treatment they will somehow magically be "fixed." They seem to hope that somehow their life will change without their having to make changes.

Recovery is a daily practice that requires effort. Anything of value requires hard work. That includes recovery. People in recovery, as in life, do not get something for nothing. That is just not how life works. Those who do the work benefit from the fruits of their work. Those who do not make the effort do not enjoy the benefits of recovery. Your life will not change for the better without your making efforts to live better.

The most important effort required of you is to work on your recovery every day. But what do you work on? I will briefly review with you some of the things you need to work on.

As discussed previously, you will likely need medication as part of your treatment. You may also need therapy to heal from trauma or other psychiatric and medical illnesses. Make sure you get all the treatment you need.

Go in to recovery with an open mind. Trust the process, because it does work.

Daniel, 38

You will then need to practice the craving and trigger management skills I discussed in earlier lessons. Go to mutual help meetings and develop recovery supports. Use your recovery supports to help you renounce addicting and manage your pain. Work on your recovery in some way, every day. Read recovery literature. Write in your recovery journal. Talk to someone about recovery every day.

You will also need to practice taking good care of yourself as described in a previous lesson. This in itself is almost a full-time job. You need to be well to fully enjoy life.

As part of this, be sure to engage in a daily spiritual practice. Practice a reverence for Reality. Pay attention to this moment—practice presence. Practice an appreciation for this gift of consciousness.

You will also need to make efforts to live a meaningful life. Your meaning will come from your devotion to a purpose that is greater than you. Live for something higher than just self-gratification. Devote yourself to a life of love. When, through your efforts, you realize a life of joy, it will be too good to give up for painkillers.

Effort requires discipline. Motivate yourself by taking accountability for your life. You are solely responsible for your success or failure. Success will be yours if you discipline yourself to make the effort. Visualize your ideal life in recovery, and then go about taking action to make your vision a reality. Live a scheduled, organized life. Take small steps and reward yourself along the way.

See life as a practice and yourself as a practitioner of life. The more you practice, the better you will get. Work daily on your recovery and your recovery will reward you with the peace, joy, and fulfillment that make the required effort well worth it!

43. Recovery is much more than just stopping painkillers.

You may think that if you just stop taking painkillers, then all will be well. If that is true for you, then you are in a small minority. For most people, and I suspect this is probably true for you as well, recovery is much more than stopping painkillers. Stopping painkillers is just the first step.

You may have started taking painkillers because you were in physical pain, emotional pain, or both. That's why they call them "painkillers." You wanted to "kill" your pain. Now that you are stopping painkillers, what will you do with your pain? If you take something away, you have to put something back in its place. What will you put back in place of the painkillers? How will you manage and hopefully resolve your pain? How will you learn to live with the inevitable pain of life without painkillers? It is your recovery that addresses these questions.

If people could recover by just stopping painkillers, then we would not have an opioid epidemic. But we do. Most likely you have tried stopping painkillers and found that "Just say 'no'" just doesn't work. If you suffer from addiction, you not only have the pain that drove you to addiction, you also have the compulsion to keep taking painkillers even when you don't want to. That is another reason why recovery is more than just stopping painkillers.

Addiction is a tricky illness. I've seen many people who just stopped taking painkillers for a period of time, sometimes for several years. But the addiction didn't go away. It just went to sleep. Then, at some later time, the addiction reemerged, again damaging the person's life. This is another reason why recovery is more than just stopping painkillers.

As mentioned earlier, you will need to address the pain that drove you to addiction in the first place. This may be physical pain, emotional pain, or both. I have patients who used opiates to deal with anger, anxiety, stress, or depression. For some patients, opiates gave them energy. Other patients were in legitimate physical pain and needed to switch to an effective non-narcotic pain management regimen. Whatever the nature of your pain, your recovery will involve treatment and support to manage and resolve it without painkillers.

Since your brain has been altered by opiates and you now suffer from addiction, you will need treatment and recovery supports to deal with compulsions and cravings. As I've discussed, you may need medications to take away cravings or to protect you if urges to addict overcome you. Medications, treatment, and recovery practices will all be a key part of your recovery.

44. Recovery changes everything in your life.

The thing that changes in recovery is everything.

There are three components to our experience of the world. First, there is how you experience Reality, or your experience of being alive. How present are you? To what degree are you lost in thought? What is your basic attitude toward the experience of being? Is it reverent, indifferent, or hostile? Does being alive feel basically positive, neutral, or negative? Do you experience grace, or do you sense that the Universe is "rigged" against you? Do you feel good and whole, or do you feel broken and unlovable? This is your way of being.

Second, there is your way of seeing the world around you. This is your understanding of yourself, others, and Reality. Do you see yourself and others as basically good, or bad? When you look at your life, do you mostly see what is not right, or what is good? Do you see life as sacred, or as meaningless? Do you understand that Reality is perfect exactly as it is, or is it flawed? Do you see that there are some basic principles by which life works best, or is it every man for himself? Do you see yourself as separate from everyone else, or do you see that you are part of a greater whole? These and other basic assumptions and understandings make up your philosophy of life, or your worldview. You may think, for example, that the best way to get by is to compete, or you may think that the best way to get by is to cooperate and collaborate. You may think that might makes right, or that it is better to live by a set of morals or virtues.

Third, there is your way of doing things. This refers to your actions, or how you behave. Do you seek immediate gratification over delayed gratification? Do you act with integrity, or do you do what you want without regard for a higher set of morals or principles? Do you live for something greater than yourself, or act only out of self-concern? Do you live solely to procure your own safety and comfort, or do you live to enhance the lives of others as well? Do you live in a way that puts you in harmony with others, or do you find yourself frequently in conflict?

Recovery entails a change in your way of being, seeing, and doing.

In recovery, you cultivate a way of being in which you experience your innate goodness and wholeness. You cultivate the capacity for presence. You develop an unconditional reverence for the gift of existence for yourself, for others, and for Reality. You develop the capacity to appreciate even the painful aspects of life and to appreciate yourself and others despite all our flaws and shortcomings. This gives you a sense of enduring peace amid the storms of life. In short, you develop a loving attitude.

In recovery, you cultivate a way of seeing in which you come to understand that Life is about Life, and not solely about you. You see that you are part of the greater whole of Life. You see your place in the order of things. You develop humility. You see that the Universe is indeed rigged in your favor, that grace exists, and that this perfectly imperfect world is sacred. You see that nothing lasts, making this moment all the more sacred. In short, you develop a loving perspective.

In recovery, you cultivate a loving way of doing things. You come into harmony with others and with the rest of Reality. You live to enhance both your life and the lives of others. You devote yourself to a greater purpose that gives your life meaning and a sense of fulfillment. You live by a higher code of love-based values. When enhancing your life and the life of others becomes what is most important to you, love becomes the central organizing principle of your life. In short, you become a loving person.

As you change your way of being, seeing, and doing, you will notice that the Universe resonates with you. It generously mirrors back the good that you put out into the world with an abundance of goodness in return. This is karma. When you are living a life of love, the pains that drove you to addiction will diminish and become quite manageable without the compulsion to addictively numb them.

45. Recovery starts with your attitude.

What is your attitude about recovery? Is recovery something you fear? Is it something you resent? Do you feel like giving up painkillers is condemning you to a joyless, miserable life? Do you feel like recovery is the best of two bad options? Or maybe it is the worst? Perhaps you feel the work required of you is too much. You may feel recovery is too much of a hassle.

You may also be feeling sorry for yourself that you are in this predicament, largely through no fault of your own. Although you chose to take painkillers, you certainly didn't choose to become addicted. You may be feeling resentful for this whole mess.

If you have a negative attitude about recovery, know that you are not alone. Negativity is a natural reaction to pain. What you are experiencing is human.

Change is difficult. Giving up an addiction is difficult. Recovery can be quite painful at times, especially during the first year or two. When you take away painkillers, putting recovery in their place can be a lot of work.

If you have a negative attitude toward recovery, know that this is where your recovery work begins. You have control over your attitude. You will not succeed in your recovery with a negative attitude, so you must change your attitude to a positive attitude.

How do you cultivate a positive attitude? Through the practice of unconditional appreciation. This will sound a little crazy, but start by appreciating your negative attitude. Have a positive attitude toward your negative attitude. See that your negativity arises out of pain and fear and nonacceptance of the way things are. Your appreciation will then trigger the experience of compassion for yourself.

Second, begin to practice an attitude of appreciation for your addiction. Appreciate that you have this "brain illness." Your attitude about recovery needs to be one of unconditional appreciation.

How do you appreciate your addiction? I suggest that you reflect carefully on the following simple truths about your situation and about recovery:

- Your addiction has brought upon you much pain. This pain can be a gift, if you will only appreciate it, not make an enemy out of it, and listen to what it is trying to tell you. Your pain gives you the opportunity to practice an attitude of unconditional appreciation for all experience, including your pain. When you appreciate your pain, you take the suffering out of distress. Then you can look closely at your pain and learn from it. What is it trying to teach you? How are you not right with Life? How do you need to change your ways of seeing, being, and doing?

- Your addiction is forcing you to now live at a higher spiritual level that will eventually bring you joy and fulfillment. You can no longer survive by numbing pain with pleasure. You now have to learn to bear pain with peace and to skillfully resolve pain as much as you can. Your addiction is forcing you to become a master at pain management. It is forcing your spiritual growth. Through recovery, you will become a wise and loving person because you must. This is the gift of your addiction.

Reflect upon the simple truth that all experience is sacred, whether painful or pleasurable. Cultivate an attitude of humble reverence for this moment. Practice an attitude of unconditional appreciation for all experience, including your recovery.

Finally, reflect upon the miracle and grace of recovery. Because of the opportunity of recovery, you are blessed. Because of recovery, your situation is not hopeless. Be grateful that effective treatments exist. Be grateful that there are so many loving people out there waiting for the opportunity to support you, to help you heal, and to help you grow. Be grateful that you have the opportunity to now embark on the most wonderful, life-changing experience of your life. Have gratitude in knowing that if you work on your recovery, you will realize a joyful and fulfilling life.

46. There are three overlapping phases of recovery.

Recovery is a progressive process over time. You will work on some things first and then on other things later. Recovery is much like building a house, where you start by digging a hole and putting in a foundation followed by building the walls and roof followed by completing the finishing touches. Just like building a house happens in phases, recovery also happens in phases.

There are three overlapping phases of recovery:

- First, you must cease addicting. This is the *renunciation* phase, in which you renounce all addicting.
- Second, heal and learn to live life skillfully. This is the *integration and repair* stage.
- The third stage is learning how to live a fulfilling life without addiction. This is the *self-realization* phase

During early recovery, you will focus primarily on renouncing all addicting. This is your first act of self-love. You must stop harming yourself before you can begin to heal. Also, you cannot learn to let go of compulsively numbing cravings by addicting unless you stop addicting.

Only then can you learn to manage and resolve cravings without addicting and address the pain that triggers your cravings in other love-based ways.

The damage to your brain's drive-reward system can make cravings and compulsions overwhelming. You will need the support of others as you practice putting the part of your brain that makes reasonable decisions back in charge of your actions. You will need to practice ways of bearing your distress, soothing yourself, and distracting yourself from your distress. Use your cravings as an opportunity to practice appreciation of your experience combined with restraint. You will also likely need to empower yourself by taking medications that help diminish cravings and compulsions.

In your middle phase of recovery, you will primarily work on healing trauma, including the traumas of your addiction. You will also need to attend to any underlying psychiatric or medical issues. You may need three to five years of therapy to do this work. You will attend to rebuilding your life and repairing the damage done by your addiction. You will work on living life skillfully, including learning to manage your pain skillfully. You will learn how to have healthy relationships. You will practice humility and integrity in all your affairs.

In the latter phase of recovery, you will begin to realize your full potential to nurture and savor Life in the ways that are unique to you. Through your daily spiritual practice, you will realize your life vision, and experience wholeness and fulfillment. It is in this final phase of recovery that you will experience an enduring joy and peace regardless of your circumstances. You will experience openness, clarity, and freedom. As you live love, the Universe will generously and lovingly resonate with you. You will be addiction-free.

47. Recovery is joyful and fulfilling.
The fruits of recovery are joy and fulfillment. When you choose to act with self-love before self-gratification, doing the next right thing results in the next right consequence. In addiction, you did what felt good regardless of what was right. Now, in recovery, you do what is right regardless of urges to feel better through addicting. As you put good out into the world, good comes back to you. This is the karma of recovery. This karma will bring you joy.

Recovery frees you from the self-destruction of addiction. When you are in recovery, you are healthy, well, living a positive, connected, and meaningful life. You experience the joy of contributing and realizing your full potential.

Recovery is a healing of what is broken in you. When you heal, you create the conditions to experience the joy that is your birthright. It is in our true nature to be joyful when our basic needs are met and we are not in pain. Recovery is joyful, because in recovery you develop effective ways of meeting your needs for safety, comfort, belonging, and, most importantly, for loving and being loved. When you meet these needs, the natural consequence is the childlike experience of joy.

What is fulfillment? The word itself seems rather vague, but here are just a few examples of what might be fulfilling: caring for a partner, caring for a child, making something new, providing a service to someone, or doing something you love, such as playing an instrument, going hiking, or playing a sport.

The possibilities of things to do that might be fulfilling for you are endless. Just think about things you enjoy doing that would be rewarding if you were to do them. Be creative. Then, think about how you could do these things in ways that might be useful to others. One example is a patient of mine who loves to clean. She works as a house cleaner and loves her work. She finds it fulfilling to leave a house fresh and clean for her clients, who love and appreciate her for the great work she does. Her life as a house cleaner is very fulfilling for her. Doing something that fulfills you gives you a life beyond simple self-gratification. What is it you are called to do? You have been given this gift of consciousness, this gift of life. Life calls upon you to nurture and savor Life in the ways that are unique to you. Look within. What are the deepest yearnings of your soul that seemingly arise from beyond you and demand expression through you? Also, look outside of yourself. What does the world ask of you? How are you asked to contribute? You can experience fulfillment in your work, in creating something, in service to others, in righting a wrong, and in caring for your family and friends. Life feels fulfilling and meaningful when in some way you have made the world a better place.

As you look within yourself and outside of yourself, you will see that there is a place where the longings of your soul and the longings of the world overlap. When you then live to fulfill these longings, you experience fulfillment.

You will not think about fulfillment while you are addicted. Trying to keep up with the demands of the addiction is not among your higher spiritual callings. When you live to serve the disease, you do not live to serve Life. If you do not live to serve Life, you will not experience fulfillment.

In recovery, you free yourself from the prison of addiction so that you can now listen to and answer the callings both from within and without. You can tend to your passions. You can cultivate your gifts. You can give. You can serve. You can grow into the unique, authentic person that you are. Recovery gives you this gift. This is why recovery is both joyful and fulfilling.

48. Recovery promotes personal growth.

When you stop hurting yourself by addicting, you create the opportunity for healing. In order to heal, you must overcome the "messages" from the part of your brain that call upon you to addict.

How do you grow emotionally in recovery? In recovery, you learn how to live life more skillfully. You learn how to take good care of yourself. You learn how to protect yourself.

You learn how to belong and contribute. Several shifts occur within you as you move from addiction into recovery. These shifts enhance your personal growth. These are positive shifts in your way of being, seeing, and doing:

- From relief-seeking to facing, embracing, and dealing with your pain
- From corruption to integrity
- From self-centered to other-oriented
- From delusion and self-deception to clarity, insight, and awareness
- From poor judgment to good judgment
- From immaturity to maturity
- From impulsivity and compulsivity to restraint and thoughtfulness
- From destructive behavior to nurturing behavior
- From dishonesty to honesty
- From self-hatred to self-love
- From taking from others to giving to others
- From deprivation to abundance
- From self-obsession to love
- From shame to healthy remorse
- From hopelessness to hope
- From negativity to appreciation
- From entitlement to gratitude
- From isolation to connection
- From inferiority to wholeness
- From empty to fulfilled
- From unaccountable to accountable

When you recover, you grow. You transform from a broken person to a beautiful person. As you transform, you will experience that your life transforms from a broken life to a beautiful life. This may seem far off to you right now. Personal growth does take time. In fact, it takes a lifetime.

On the other hand, you can start right now, where you are, by renouncing addicting, asking for help, getting treatment, taking good care of yourself, and doing the next right thing. Growth involves acting your way into feeling whole. If you just take care of this moment, you will slowly grow and transform. Be patient. Persist. Have hope. A better future is awaiting you.

49. Recovery is the practice of love.
Recovery is the practice of love. Love for self, love for others, and love for life. What is love? First, love is not a feeling. It is much deeper than that. Love is two things. It is an attitude of reverence for Life followed by actions to enhance Life.

The attitude of love is one of an unconditional reverence for this miraculous gift of existence and for the Life that sustains us and of which we are a part. It is a reverence for the Now. When I say this attitude is unconditional, I mean that it persists beneath the ever-changing swirl of feelings and mood states that we experience from moment to moment. This includes the pain, negativity, and cravings of addiction. As I discussed earlier, you start your recovery with the practice of loving appreciation and reverence for your life as it is right now, in the midst of the pain of your addiction.

A loving attitude of reverence for Life inspires our devotion to act to enhance life. Love is thus a serious, committed endeavor. In love, we live for the One Life that sustains us and of which we are a part. When you practice love, you refrain from harming Life—including your life—in everything you say and do. Love is a combination of abstaining from destructive behavior and taking action to make things better—for yourself and others. Out of your reverence for Life, you practice asking yourself, "What would love do?" moment-by-moment.

As you love yourself and others in all that you say and do, you experience the consequences of love. When you love yourself, you enhance your vitality. When you stop harming yourself, you feel better. You see that practicing love is good for you.

When you were addicting, you had the intention to love, in that you were addicting to feel better. Your love was unskillful and unwise, however, because it did not enhance your life. Acting on urges to feel better and not feel bad are not always loving. Sometimes, as with addiction, our actions make things worse. Love requires wisdom and clarity. When we act with love, we do what is best for everyone regardless of urges to do otherwise that may give temporary relief. In love, you refrain from immediate gratification or relief if you see that this will cause you or others harm. This is why abstaining from destructive action is just as important as taking constructive action.

When you love others, you feel more lovable. As you do what is right, you begin to feel right. Integrity—or doing the next right thing—is a core practice of love. There are other love practices that make up the practice of recovery. They are:

- Accountability
- Affirmation
- Assertiveness
- Authenticity
- Caution
- Charity
- Compassion
- Consideration
- Courage
- Devotion
- Discipline
- Empathy
- Endurance
- Forgiveness
- Gratitude
- Helpfulness
- Hope
- Humility
- Kindness
- Nurturing
- Patience
- Trustworthiness
- Wisdom

In your recovery, you practice living these virtues in your everyday life. As you engage in these love practices, your life flowers. It is through the practice of love that you will optimize your vitality and realize the full measure of the joy that life has to offer you.

50. Joy will protect you from readdicting.

When you engage in the practice of recovery, you engage in the practice of love. When you engage in the practice of love, you experience the consequences of loving. The consequences of loving are joy and fulfillment.

When you are full of joy, your cravings to addict with painkillers—or with any other substance for that matter—

subside. Joy serves as a buffer against cravings. When you are full of joy, you feel that your life is just too good to give up for the temporary high of a painkiller. In your clarity, you see that the temporary relief or pleasure of addicting is not worth the long-term consequences of addicting. You experience that joy is much better than addicting.

I learned that being honest and transparent in living your life is really an important part of recovery. If you start telling lies again, the addiction circles right back around.

Susan, 38

Addiction is driven by pain or the lack of joy. If you are in pain, you addict to numb your pain. If you suffer from a lack of joy, you feel a vague sense of boredom or emptiness. You feel a yearning for "something more." This lack of joy is a spiritual pain, because you are cut off from the experience of wonder and awe inspired by the simple fact of your miraculous existence. When you are spiritually awake, resting in the experience of stillness, love, compassion, and joy naturally arise. Joy is a natural byproduct of your spiritual vitality.

When you are full of joy, you don't experience the cravings for "something more." Like a ray of light, joy casts out the darkness of emptiness in your consciousness. This moment is then far more than enough. There is no need to enhance it with painkillers or other consciousness-altering substances and behaviors.

When you are full of joy, your relationship to your pain changes. In your recovery, you will develop an underlying attitude of joy that persists below and along with your negative emotional states. You may be sad, angry, hurt, afraid, or in physical pain. When you are, your joy will protect you.

Joy changes your relationship to your pain. With joy, pain is no longer an enemy you must either kill or flee from. With joy, you can face and embrace your pain. Joy enables you to live with unavoidable pain. Joy also enables you to work through and resolve pain that can be resolved. Joy is the bedrock upon which you stand as you engage in the experience of Life.

If a loved one leaves you or dies, you will naturally feel tremendous sadness, grief, and perhaps anger. This is natural. You will be in great pain. When this happens, your joy will help to protect you from addicting. Your joy puts your pain in its proper perspective. Joy helps you maintain your loving attitude toward life. Out of your love for Life, you resolve to bear and resolve your pain with love rather than by addicting. In this way, your joy carries you through the dark periods of life.

51. There are many ways to cultivate joy.
You will cultivate your joy in your recovery through intentional practices. Effort—gentle, persistent effort—is required. The following twenty "joy practices" will help you to savor the gift of your existence.

- *Stop hurting yourself.* Renounce addicting. Protect yourself as you go about your day. Be careful so as to minimize harm to yourself and others. Remember that Life feeds on Life, and that evil exists. Just as Life sustains you, so, too, can it consume you. Take care and do nothing to bring harm upon yourself. Renounce destructive habits. Instead commit to caring for yourself as a parent cares for their cherished child.

- *Let go and forgive.* Stop resenting Reality—the people in your life and the conditions of your life—for not conforming to your ideas of how things should be. Be humble. See that Life is about Life, and not just about you. Release old hurts, resentments, and judgments. Replace negative judgments with discernment. Seek to understand, as understanding breeds compassion.

- *Get still.* Engage in a spiritual practice of silence, solitude, and stillness. Your practice could be meditation, prayer, or contemplation. Mind-body practices such as yoga are also an option. Through your stillness practice, you will cultivate your reverence and respect for Reality. In stillness, you can calm your mind. You allow yourself to experience the ease and peace of being. Your stillness then becomes a refuge from the mind-made pains of life.

- *Practice presence.* As you go through your day, practice presence. Make a gentle effort to be still while still moving. Cultivate "beginner's mind," savoring each moment as if it were both your first and last moment. Cultivate inquisitiveness. Look and listen so you can see deeply and hear deeply.

- *Keep it fresh.* Be open. Recognize the grace and abundance that are all around you. Let stillness be your anchor and refuge. You will cultivate inner peace through your practice of stillness. The practice of presence will cultivate loving kindness and joy. In still presence, attend fully to every joyful experience, starting with the simple joy of taking a breath.

- *Savor existence.* Start each day with an intention to savor all the simple joys of life. Savor the ability to see, to hear, to feel, to taste, and to touch. Savor the beauty that is all around you. Savor the miracle of your existence.

- *Practice self-love.* As you practice reverence for the Now, take particular care to practice self-reverence. This may be difficult if you were neglected, unloved, or harmed growing up. If this is the case, you will need to engage in a daily intentional practice of self-love. Accept your fears, your faults, your misdeeds and mistakes, and your negativity bias. See that your brain, and not you, generates your thoughts, feelings, and urges based upon previous and present conditions.

- *Stop taking yourself personally.* Paradoxically, change begins with reverent self-acceptance, self-compassion, and self-forgiveness. Be kind to yourself while holding yourself accountable for your actions.

- *Heal.* Get treatment for medical and psychiatric conditions. If you have been broken by neglect or trauma, get help to heal and discover your wholeness. Practice all of these joy practices daily, as they, too, will help you to heal.

- *Take care.* Take good care of yourself. Live life skillfully and intelligently. Eat well, sleep, rest, exercise, and engage in a daily spiritual practice. Your joy will flower from your vitality.

- *Manage pain with love.* Manage your pain with love rather than with attempting to numb yourself. Soothe yourself with controlled deep breaths and other calming mind-body practices. Comfort yourself with positive affirmations and reassurances. Replace addicting with connecting.

- *Ask for help and support.* See that love is all around you if you only reach out and ask for help. Get connected and avoid isolation.

- *Practice respectful authenticity.* Be who you are. Have the courage to be you. Let yourself experience the vulnerability of authenticity. Don't take others' nonacceptance or condemnations of you personally. Practice unconditional self-love even in the face of others' criticisms or condemnations. Remember that unconditional love goes both ways. Remind yourself that if you act with love and integrity, that you have done your part, and that others' reactions are not about you—they are about them. When you make mistakes—which you will do every day of your life—forgive yourself for being perfectly imperfect. Show yourself the love and compassion you deserve, even when others do not.

- *Have fun.* Play. Do what you love. Make time for simple pleasures. Savor the small things that can bring joy, like a meal, a walk around the block, the smile and laugh of a friend, or a warm shower. Watch the sunrise or sunset. Be in nature. Enjoy music and the arts. Sing. Be creative. Hang out. Balance doing and being. Read a good book. Dance. Relax. Take a nap. Watch a movie. Slow down.

- *Be with joyful others.* Be with positive, joyful people doing positive, joyful things. Be with those you love. Maintain connection rituals and routines, such as family dinners and social events with friends.

- *Be grateful.* Practice gratitude—for life, for love, and for abundance. Notice what is good in your life. Focus on the many good things, not the few distressing things. Say thank you.

- *Practice loving.* Start each day with an intention to love. As you go through your day, practice compassion—especially self-compassion—empathy, generosity, contentedness, hopefulness, appreciation, humility, patience, forgiveness, and kindness. Be helpful. Yield to others' needs out of loving mutuality. Cultivate an unconditional friendliness toward yourself and others. Wish yourself and others peace, happiness, and joy. Love Life. As you love, so will Life resonate with your loving. You will realize the joy of making a difference to others and will experience love coming back to you many times over.

- *Practice positivity.* See the opportunities in difficult situations. Your reverence for this moment will lead to a positive attitude, which will lead to positive thoughts, which will result in positive actions, which will lead to positive outcomes.

- *Seek out humor.* Enjoy comedy. Laugh often. Practice smiling on purpose—it will make you feel better.

- *Live with balance.* We live out of balance in a culture that prizes doing and achievement above all. In our rush to do, do, do, we lose our opportunity to savor Life. Simply being is greatly underrated. Balance doing and being. Balance work, love, and play. Remember that love and play are more important than work.

- *Visualize joy.* Recall past moments of joy. Remember yourself as a child having fun. Bring the feeling of past experiences of joy into this present moment.

- *Discover.* Cultivate the joy of discovery. Make learning and growth a life habit. Practice an art, such as playing an instrument, sculpting, or drawing. Take classes. Read books. Listen closely to others and ask questions. Strive to understand.

- *Live a meaningful life.* Take at least one action a day toward your higher goals and dreams. Live for the One Life of which you are a part. When you live for your higher purpose, you cultivate the joy of meaning.

The time to experience joy is right now, as you begin your recovery work. There is no need to wait for a certain set of circumstances. You have a choice. Just as you can choose recovery, so can you choose to engage in these practices of joy.

52. A higher purpose will serve you well.

Why do you live? Why do you do what you do? Why do you eat? If you look closely at these questions, you will see that you have more than one purpose for living. You have a basic purpose and a higher purpose.

Your basic purpose is to survive and pass on your genes to the next generation if that is your choice. This is Life's core mandate. Life has designed you and equipped you with an ego in order to ensure your survival and so that you can procreate. Your ego drives you to act in ways to secure your safety, comfort, and status as a member of your family and community. Your ego is all about feeling good and not feeling bad. It is about gratification, whether it be sexual gratification, the gratification of a good meal, or the gratification of being respected, appreciated, admired, or feared by others. Out of concern for your survival, your ego is concerned with power and control.

We humans also have a higher purpose, which also enhances our survival as a species. That purpose is to love. It is to nurture Life and to savor this gift of existence.

Although the ego (your sense of self, or "I," "me," or "mine") is a necessary survival system, it can lead us astray if it is not in service to our higher purpose. For the ego, there is never enough safety, comfort, or status. This moment is never enough. Imagine you win the lottery and travel to Tahiti. You are in an island paradise and enjoying yourself tremendously.

However, after a few days or weeks, you get used to your new life. Your ego will have you complaining about the heat or the bugs. You will find yourself forever wanting for something more. This is why your ego lies at the root of your addiction. Since for the ego this moment is never enough, there is always the craving for something more. That craving turns to an addictive substance or behavior when you suffer from an addiction.

I've learned to let things go, to let other people's crap go by me. I continue on in life doing what I need to do and stay focused. Recovery allows me to stay focused.

Robert, 34

Let's imagine that you are a carpenter. You are working on building a house. Why are you building this house? Is it to make money so you can eat, secure a place to live, and have some money for entertainment? If so, these are legitimate reasons for doing what you are doing. They serve your basic purpose.

Perhaps you are also building this house to make money to support your family. There is a part of you that wants to take care of people you love. Perhaps you are also building this house for the fulfillment of providing another family a place to live. These motivations serve your higher purpose.

Even though your basic purpose brings gratification, your higher purpose brings fulfillment. Your higher purpose makes building a house meaningful. When you live for your higher purpose, you experience the joy of meaning. You experience the joy of loving. Unlike the pleasure of gratification, which lasts for but a moment, the joy of loving lasts a lifetime. When you live for your higher purpose, there is no need for "something more." This moment is more than enough. This is why living for the higher purpose of loving protects you from addicting.

Begin every day with an intention to love. This is your higher purpose. If you live to love, with your ego in service to this higher purpose, you will experience the joy, fulfillment, and abundance that will protect you from falling back into addicting.

53. Learn to have fun.

Recovery is part work, part love, and part play. A life of recovery is a life of balance in which play revitalizes you. Make it an intention to have fun every day. Make time to let the child inside of you come out to play. Successful people in life and in recovery get more done in less time by devoting part of each day to having fun. They take time each day to play. You should do the same.

Fun and play are good for you. Having fun is something you do for its own sake, not for a particular outcome. Play engages you so that you lose yourself in having fun. Fun serves your need to savor Life and helps to relieve stress. Play helps you to laugh, which brightens your mood and enhances your vitality.

You will need breaks in your recovery from the seriousness of life. Having fun will help to sustain you through the stresses of survival, renew you, and keep you from becoming dull. Play will keep you young at heart. It may even prolong your life. It will help fuel your joy, which will keep your cravings to addict at bay.

Having fun fuels creativity and enhances mood. Ironically, it can actually help you solve problems by taking you away from those problems for a while. When you play with others, you deepen, heal, and revitalize your relationships.

The ways to have fun are endless:

- Reading for fun
- Playing a sport
- Engaging in a hobby
- Solving puzzles
- Going to the movies
- Listening to music
- Practicing an art; taking an art class
- Going to parties and entertaining
- Going to museums and performances
- Joking, telling stories
- Going to comedy shows

- Playing board and card games
- Going on outings and trips
- Visiting new places; sightseeing; exploring
- Playing video games
- Playing with children
- Joining a singing group
- Going out with friends to sporting events, go bowling, play miniature golf, or join in some other fun group activity

Make having fun an active, not passive activity. Avoid zoning out in front of the TV. Instead, do things that engage you. Don't make play anything more than play. If you get too competitive, the purpose of winning takes over. If you practice an art as play, allow yourself to just enjoy yourself without focusing on perfection.

Just as you budget time for work and love, budget time for play. Take advantage of opportunities to have fun, such as joking with strangers while waiting in line at the grocery store. Make time every day for a little play. Make time each week for a special outing or activity. Mix it up, adding novelty and variety to your play. This breaks up the routines that can become ruts.

Having fun serves as a powerful antidote to cravings. You will want to schedule fun time into every day if at all possible. Work, love, and play in healthy portions every day.

54. Learn to be appreciative.

You have control over only three things in life: what you pay attention to, your attitude, and your actions. I have already touched on the importance of a positive attitude toward your recovery. The most useful attitude is an attitude of unconditional appreciation of your experience, even if it is painful. Appreciation is far better than non-appreciation, for non-appreciation fuels suffering, which fuels addiction.

Appreciating the positive in your life will enhance your joy, which will protect you from readdicting. Take a daily inventory of all that is good in your life. This is the practice of gratitude, or counting your blessings. Start with an appreciation of the gift of Awareness. You are a part of the Universe and you are aware. How amazing, mysterious, and miraculous this is. Savor this incredible gift of self-aware consciousness. Then consider the gifts of air to breath; water to drink; the sun that gives light, energy, and life to this planet; and the rich earth. Reflect on the gifts of being able to see, hear, walk, feel, and think. Then consider the gifts of food, clothing, and shelter.

Also, appreciate your friends and family and the many people available to help you in your healing and recovery. Appreciate your talents and achievements. Appreciate the innumerable gifts of human civilization and the abundant and generous web of life that sustains you. Think of the millions of people who all contributed in some way to your ability to live this long and to being able to read this book. If you reflect just a little on this, you will feel a profound appreciation for humanity, for those who have loved you along the way, and for the innumerable contributions of millions of other people to your life.

Then there is the appreciation of pain. This is not to say that you should enjoy being in pain. No one enjoys being in pain. Pain is something to be avoided, minimized, and endured. Yet pain brings gifts, and merits your appreciation. Take, for example, the pain of addiction. Pain is your teacher, telling you that you are not living in harmony with Life and Reality in ways that enhance your well-being. Your addictive cravings and compulsions are signals that your brain is not working properly and needs your tending through the process of recovery. The pain of your addiction forces you to grow, to live life more skillfully, and to live on a higher plane out of love. Your addiction forces you to grow spiritually into a beautiful human being. For these reasons, your addiction is something to be appreciated.

There are numerous other pains of existence, both internal and external. These include poverty, hunger, war, exploitation, neglect, abuse, physical illness, anxiety, depression, trauma, self-hatred, shame, fatigue, anxiety, anger, sadness, and grief. There is the sad reality that life is not permanent. Each day we live is one day less that we have to live on this planet. The realization of this can be very painful.

Finally, there is the appreciation of grace, forgiveness, and healing. You are a loving and intelligent being living in a loving and intelligent Universe. This is an appreciation for the reality and power of love. When you reflect in this way, you will see that you are truly, profoundly blessed. You will realize that this moment of precious existence is sacred.

Engage in a persistent, patient practice of appreciation for all of life's pains. They all serve as impersonal guides and teachers. They signal to you that you are somehow not right with Reality and that there is a need for change in either your attitude, your circumstances, or both. Listen appreciatively to your pain. Do what you can to ease your pain. For the pains and discomforts you cannot relieve, practice appreciative acceptance and allowance.

Practice letting go of your compulsion to make Reality other than what it is. In this way, even senseless and unavoidable pain can be your spiritual teachers. The practice of appreciation gives you the gifts of peace, serenity, freedom, and compassion—both for yourself and for all those who suffer as you have suffered. Appreciating your pain will strengthen your resilience and help you to both endure and savor this gift of existence despite your pain.

55. Practice good self-care.

The basic truth of recovery is that you can only "do good if you are good." You will need to optimize your vitality in order to have a vital, successful recovery.

Recovery is hard work. Recovery requires effort. Recovery will be more difficult for you if you do not feel well. You need to take good care of yourself in order to feel well.

You are a dynamic living system that requires continuous maintenance and care to survive and to fully function. You need to tend to your vitality every day in order to sustain it. You are the one who is responsible for taking good care of yourself. While we all need the help of others to get by in life, you alone are accountable for your well-being.

Make a life commitment right now to being your own ideal parent. Commit to taking very good care of yourself as if you were your own cherished child. If you truly, completely commit to loving yourself in all that you say and do, you will both protect yourself fiercely from being harmed by others and you will also do nothing to harm yourself in any way, including by addicting. You will also do whatever you must to enhance and maintain your well-being, including doing things that you may not feel like doing, because they are what is best for you. This is where the loving practices of self-discipline and self-control come in. This is being a good parent to yourself.

Taking good care of yourself means asking for help along the way. No one lives life or does recovery alone. Humbly recognize your needs and vulnerabilities. Let others help you.

Take good care of yourself by eating healthful foods. Don't poison your system with processed foods just because they are convenient or taste good. A good parent would not do this to their child.

Take good care of yourself by getting plenty of rest. A good parent does not allow their child to become sleep-deprived.

Take good care of yourself by keeping regular routines. A good parent makes sure their child goes to bed and gets up at the same times every day. A good parent makes sure their child eats on a regular schedule.

Take good care of yourself by exercising. You need exercise to stay healthy and to feel your best. Make sure you exercise even if you don't really feel like doing so.

Take good care of yourself by having fun and playing. Also, engage in a daily spiritual practice. Soothe yourself when you are hurting with loving self-compassion and kindness.

If you parent yourself well, you will feel well. If you feel well, you will do well in your recovery. Your life is precious. See this. Also see that you have only this one precious life to live, and that each day it grows one day shorter. Seeing the preciousness of your life, commit to taking very, very good care of yourself.

56. Learn to relax.

You will need to build in rest and relaxation as part of your recovery. Relaxation rejuvenates. If you only work, you will burn yourself out. Part of taking good care of yourself includes taking breaks and relaxing.

Relaxation has many benefits. They include:

- Reducing muscle tension and pain
- Reducing stress hormones
- Improving digestion
- Lowering blood pressure
- Restoring your energy
- Reducing anxiety—promoting a feeling of calm and confidence
- Enhancing creativity
- Improving your ability to cope
- Improving insomnia
- Reducing cravings to addict

When you relax, you feel better. When you feel better, you will feel less pain. When you feel less pain, you will be less likely to experience cravings to addict to numb your pain.

Build in daily relaxation exercises into your daily routine. These might include such activities as:

- *Controlled deep breathing.* Breathe deeply in while slowly counting to four, hold your breath for four counts, slowly breathe out for four counts, and rest for four counts before your next breath. This exercise will reduce anxiety, slow your heart rate, and stabilize your blood pressure.

- *Meditation.* Be still and practice paying attention to some aspect of this present moment. It might be your breath. You might cycle your focus from your breath to what you see, what you hear, what you feel, and to thoughts and feelings that arise, returning to your breath. You can recite a mantra or a chant. You can even practice meditation while walking or running, paying careful attention to the movement of your body.

- *Yoga.* Yoga is a mind-body practice that combines postures with breathing exercises. Yoga relaxes and tones both the mind and the body.

- *Tai chi or qigong.* These practices involve slow, mindful movements with deep breathing.

- *Progressive muscle relaxation.* This practice involves tensing and then relaxing your muscles. You can start with your toes and then gradually and slowly move up your body to your head.

- *Visualization.* Close your eyes and imagine being in a serene and beautiful place. Sense what it feels like to be present and relaxed in this refuge from your stressful life. Let your mind calm as your visualization replaces stressful thoughts.

- *A slow walk in nature.* Taking a relaxed walk in nature can really calm the mind, help you to reset your perspective on things, and rejuvenate your spirits.

As you practice mindfulness throughout your day, take note of when you feel stressed, anxious, agitated, or fatigued. When you have these feelings, take a break to relax. Even if you just take one minute to take four deep, mindful breaths, you will notice you feel better. Use these relaxation exercises to maintain your experience of calm, centered awareness throughout your day. You will not only protect your recovery, you will find that your days go better overall.

57. Emotional pain can be your greatest teacher.

I talked about appreciating pain in the lesson on appreciation. Let's talk more about the value of pain. It was pain that drove you to addict. Perhaps you took painkillers to numb these various pains. When you addicted to numb your pain, you made two mistakes. One, you failed to really investigate your pain in order to learn how you were not right with Life. Second, you failed to change either your attitude or the way you were living in order to bear and hopefully resolve your pain.

In your recovery, you will need to change your attitude toward your pain. One way to do this is to reflect on all the benefits of pain as a stern but invaluable teacher. The pain of living to serve your addiction, for example, is nature's way of helping you to wake up to the reality that addiction does not work. Pain teaches you what not to do so that you do not continue to harm yourself by addicting. Your pain helps you to wake up to see a better way—the way of recovery. By facing, enduring, and learning from your pain, your pain transforms you into a more skillful and loving person.

Emotional pain is actually your best friend. Not only can it save your life, it teaches you life's greatest lessons. If you have suffered the pain of trauma, for example, your pain teaches you compassion and forgiveness. Pain teaches you wisdom, as it forces you to reflect deeply on life. Pain also fosters your strength to endure and your resilience. Pain forces you to do what you must to heal and grow.

As you look back on your life, you will likely notice that many times of the most growth and transformation were also times of great pain. We are creatures of habit. Nature designed us not to change if everything is going well. When things are not going well, your pain forces you to change and grow. Pain is nature's way of forcing you to adapt to an ever-changing environment.

Do not make an enemy out of your pain. If you do, your pain will defeat you. You will not resolve your pain by running from it or numbing it. Nothing will change. If anything, your unaddressed pain will only worsen. Life will not get better, and you will not grow, until you face, embrace, and resolve your pain by changing your attitude, changing your behavior, or both.

It is natural and human to want to escape from pain. No one wants to hurt. You will need to intentionally override your "brain's urges," in order to face and embrace your pain. It is an act of intention to endure your pain and work it through. Motivate yourself in this effort by reassuring yourself that it is good to feel your pain while practicing loving ways of soothing yourself and resolving your pain. Practice appreciating your pain and allowing it to teach you how to live more skillfully. Be humble. Allow your pain to teach you. If you learn from your pain, you will grow. As you grow, you will live more skillfully. As you live more skillfully, you will enhance your vitality. As you enhance your vitality, you will secure your recovery.

58. Failure is your friend.

If you're like most people, you probably think that failing makes you a failure. This is not true. Actually, failure can make you a success. How can that be? You probably don't remember when you were learning to walk. As you learned, you fell down over and over again. It was in the falling and getting back up that you eventually succeeded in walking. You learned how to walk by falling down.

Now imagine you are trying to learn to ride a unicycle. It is in the falling off the unicycle that you eventually learn to keep your balance. Life, and recovery for that matter, are like this. Successful people are the ones who learned from their mistakes and kept on trying until they got it right. This is why failure is actually success in disguise. It is in your failures that you will learn life's greatest lessons.

You will experience failures in your recovery. No one does recovery perfectly. You will have many small failures, such as letting life get temporarily out of balance. You may have some big failures, such as a full-blown relapse. If you do, embrace failure as your friend. Learn from your mistakes. Let them teach you how to live more skillfully. Be humble. Get back up, brush yourself off, and persist. When you fail, say to yourself, "This is an opportunity to learn and grow."

Thomas Edison, who invented the light bulb, did just this. It's said he tried thousands of filaments before he finally found one that would light up and stay lit. Every time he failed, he reportedly would say that he had succeeded in finding yet another way to not make a light bulb. It was this positive attitude combined with perseverance that made him one of the world's greatest inventors.

Recovery requires taking risks. The biggest mistake you can make is being afraid of making mistakes. Take the risks you need to take by doing the things you've never done before. That is how you grow. You will need to do this to secure your recovery.

Many people give up when they fail. It is only in giving up that failing becomes true failure. Commit to yourself that you will be one of the successful people who honors the inevitable pain of failure not as a message to give up but as a motivator to go on. With this attitude, you are sure to have a successful recovery.

59. Recovery takes practice.

Getting really good at anything requires about 10,000 hours of practice. That's the equivalent of working forty hours a week for nearly five years. After that, people get better and better at whatever they are practicing. This is true whether it's learning to play the violin, shooting free throws, or living a joyful life free of addiction.

You may not have thought of your life as something to practice. Much of it may seem routine. You might be asking yourself, "What is there to practice?"

The answer is "Everything." There is always the opportunity to practice being mindfully present, even when you are brushing your teeth. There is always the opportunity to practice an attitude of appreciation for the gift of your life. Whenever you talk with someone, there is always the opportunity to practice treating them with reverence and respect.

If you want to get really good at recovery, you will need to practice the skills of recovery every day. You will need to be consistent and persistent. You will need to be disciplined about it. You will need to be intentional about it, living your life on purpose. If you practice, you will get better and better. After about three to five years of practice, you will probably achieve a consistently stable and joyful life free of addiction. You will need to be patient, however. The fruits of practice don't come overnight. Change takes time and repetition.

But what do you practice? You will need to practice the following recovery skills:

- Abstaining from acting on cravings to addict and resolving your cravings
- Avoiding triggers to readdict
- Managing triggers when they occur without readdicting
- Asking for help from safe and helpful people
- Recognizing humbly that you are no better or worse than anyone else, and that you have needs and need help just like everyone else

- Connecting with others respectfully and authentically
- Taking very good care of yourself
- Connecting with something greater than yourself. This could be your Higher Power, your family, your friends, your community, your recovery program, your pet, or even nature.
- Living your life for that something that is greater than yourself. This could be living to care for your family, your friends, your community, and/or for others suffering from addiction. It could also be living to create something useful through your work, or serving others in need. This is when you will shift from living for personal gratification to living for the fulfillment of loving. It is in the practice of living for something greater than yourself—in living for others—that you will ultimately heal and free yourself from the bonds of addiction.

Recovery is hard work. If you expect others to fix you, you will readdict. The good news is that recovery works if you practice at it. The bad news—though it's not really bad news—is that you have to practice recovery for recovery to work.

60. You will need commitment and discipline to stay in recovery.

You will need commitment and discipline for your recovery. Discipline is good for you. Through discipline you will realize success in your recovery. Discipline does require effort, mostly to do what is best even though you may not feel like it. It will take discipline, for example, to not act on urges to addict and to pick up the phone to talk out your cravings even when you don't feel like it.

So how can you increase your discipline? Here are some practices:

- Motivate yourself to be disciplined by seeing that a lack of discipline hurts you. See the benefits of living a disciplined life. See that discipline ultimately brings success and joy.
- Get clear about why you are committing to your recovery. What will the rewards be?

- Make a recovery plan and keep to it. If you plan to go to a meeting, go. If you plan to talk to your recovery mentor to get current, do it. Be disciplined about not letting life get in the way of your recovery.

- Every morning, visualize yourself doing what you need to do and then visualize how good you will feel when you do it.

- Look at yourself in the mirror each morning and recite your intentions for the day. Setting intentions increases your likelihood of acting on your intentions.

- Take accountability for your life. See that you are solely responsible for your circumstances and successes. See that by living a disciplined life of love and integrity you have the power to realize a joyful and fulfilling life.

- Break your recovery down into small, doable steps. Make one change at a time, gradually building up new positive life habits.

- Schedule your life. Then be firm but flexible in keeping a schedule.

- Reward yourself for your discipline. Treat yourself when you accomplish something difficult.

- Get comfortable with discomfort. Life entails distress. Your discipline will ask of you to do uncomfortable things, such as going to a meeting when you are tired or exercising when you feel like sleeping in. Doing new and difficult things is always uncomfortable at first. Expect and welcome discomfort as you discipline yourself to do what you need to do to recover.

- Make yourself accountable by recruiting accountability partners. Tell people what you intend to do and then ask them to hold you accountable for doing it.

- Get support and guidance from wise and supportive people. If you are having a hard time with discipline, ask for help.

- Don't give up. If you have difficulty with discipline, recommit to trying again and again, day after day.

Discipline is like a muscle that grows stronger with practice.

See that, rather than discipline making you miserable, your discipline will help to bring you joy. Embrace living a disciplined life as a loving thing to do for yourself and as something that will be necessary for your successful recovery.

61. Recovery requires hope and faith.

You will strengthen your commitment to recovery by strengthening your faith and hope.

Do you lack faith in yourself? You may lack faith if you've experienced a lot of physical or emotional trauma in the past. Faith can be difficult if you've met with repeated failures in the past. If others have told you that you are hopeless, you may lack hope for yourself.

Do not believe the feeling that you are hopeless. It is not true. Sometimes our feelings do not reflect reality. If you just look around you at any recovery meeting, you will find many people who suffered from severe addiction who are living beautiful lives of recovery. If they can do it, so can you. Surround yourself with these inspiring people so that they might inspire you.

If you look carefully, you will see that despite whatever misfortune you have experienced, there is also the reality of grace, resilience, healing, beauty, goodness, and love. These are yours to be had through the practice of recovery. While evil and destruction exist, see that goodness is greater, and always prevails sooner or later. See that there is a spirit of love that pervades the Universe. This spirit gave you life and continues to sustain you. This same spirit will now heal you through the practice of recovery.

Believe in your capacity to succeed. You have already succeeded in innumerable ways, or you wouldn't be reading these pages. Just as you have succeeded in getting this far in life, so can you succeed in your recovery if you work at it and persevere.

Hope is self-fulfilling. If you have hope for yourself, you will be more likely to take action to recover. Time and again, experience shows that successful people are those who believed they could succeed. Believe in your capacity to succeed. If you think you can recover, you can.

Don't let fear and hopelessness overcome you. You are not a victim of this addiction or your circumstances. Have faith that success comes not from the cards you are dealt, but from how you play those cards. If you resolve to succeed, you will succeed. If you don't believe, make believe. Fake it until you make it.

If you lack hope, borrow the hope of others. Let their hope for you sustain you and light the flame of hope within you. Don't let past mistakes and failures define you. The past only predicts the future if you let it. Let go of the past. Instead, vow to live each moment fresh, wisely, and skillfully to create a better future. You are not doomed, no matter how low you feel. Recovery is real. It is yours if you only do the work required.

You can handle whatever hardships you encounter. You need only say "Yes" to this moment and do the next right thing to soothe yourself and improve your circumstances.

Break the dream of recovery down into small, daily steps. Then just take the step before you, with faith that just taking the next step will eventually bring you to your dreams.

Recovery works for everyone who works it. That includes you. You are no different. See this, and have hope and faith that you, too, will recover to live a fulfilling life.

62. Recovery takes patience.

Recovery requires patience. Practice patience, especially with yourself. Nothing of true greatness happens overnight. This is also true of your recovery. Your recovery will take time. It takes time to heal. It takes time to learn a new way of being in the world. It takes time to discover the deeper truths of how life works. It takes time to learn how to put your newfound experience and understanding into action. As I mentioned in the lesson on practice, developing your recovery skills will take thousands of hours of practice. This will take time. You will heal, but you will need to be patient. It will not happen overnight.

You will benefit best from a "slow recovery." Make "Slow but sure" your motto. Be like the tortoise. Success comes not to the swift. It comes to those who keep patiently practicing the skills of recovery over a sustained period of time.

Everything takes time. Just as you can't make a tree grow overnight, so you cannot rush recovery. Just as it takes nine months to make a baby, so it will take several years to make a full recovery. It will take time for you to create a stable and fulfilling life free from addiction.

Although you cannot speed up the process of recovery, you can slow it down by becoming impatient and giving up. Do not get discouraged when you hit roadblocks, plateaus, or even setbacks. These are all part of the process of growth. Be patient. You will not speed up your growth by giving up.

Think how many years it took you to get to where you are right now in your life. Think about all the changes you must make in your way of being, seeing and doing, all the healing that must occur, and all the changes you wish for in your circumstances. Does it not make sense that these changes will take time? There is a saying that if you walk ten miles into the woods, you have to walk ten miles to get out. Be patient with yourself as you walk the path of recovery out of the woods of your addiction.

Just as you must be patient with yourself, so, too, must you be patient with others. Many people have likely been damaged by your addiction. Just as you need time to recover, they will also need time to recover. People need to go through their own journeys in their own way as they heal and learn to support you in your recovery. Be patient with others as well.

Patience truly is a virtue. When you are patient, you align yourself with the ebb and flow of life. Your patience will bring you into harmony with the natural unfolding of life. This will reduce the unnecessary suffering caused by impatience and help to sustain you through the ups and downs of your recovery.

63. Recovery requires perseverance.

Recovery requires perseverance. You have many challenges ahead of you. That is just the nature of life. You will have days when you feel like giving up. There will be days when your pain will feel too great to bear. You will likely experience attacks of "F*** it," in which you will want to addict and just won't care about what happens to you. Do not listen to this inner voice. When you feel you can't take another step, you must revive your strength to carry on. You will need to persevere. Let me give you some food for thought that will hopefully help you when you've lost the strength to carry on.

Know that those who persevere in their recovery are the ones who succeed in their recovery. The same holds true for life in general. Like someone once said, "The big shots are only the little shots who kept shooting." The winners are the losers who lost, but kept trying, over and over again.

You will not succeed in your recovery by giving up. You will succeed by getting up. If you find yourself readdicting—and many people do experience this—you will need to recommit and keep working at your recovery, learning from your mistakes along the way. There is a Japanese proverb that goes, "Fall seven times, stand up eight." This means that you should keep getting up and keep trying when you fall down. This is the perseverance of recovery.

When you feel like you are going through hell, keep going. Know that even the darkest of times eventually give way to the light of day. If you just persevere, the most painful days of your recovery will pass. They always do.

The mind is a powerful thing. You are capable of far more than you know. I once was backpacking up a mountain. It was the first day. I was out of shape. The trail was all uphill. My pack was heavy. After about four hours, I was tired and wanted to stop. But we were only halfway to the campsite. I didn't think I could make it the rest of the way. Fortunately or unfortunately, I had no choice. I had to hike up the rest of the mountain.

The next six hours were difficult to say the least. They were painful. I was exhausted. But I made it because I had to. I simply put one step in front of the other and kept going despite my pain. I persevered and did something I thought was impossible.

Life and recovery are like that. If you commit and believe in yourself, you are truly capable not only of recovering, but also of accomplishing great things. You have this power, if only you keep on keepin' on. This is the power of perseverance.

64. Let life's challenges strengthen you.

You might be looking at the work ahead of you and be feeling intimidated. Managing your pain without painkillers may seem nearly impossible. You have so much to accomplish to achieve a good life in recovery. The challenges ahead of you may feel overwhelming.

The truth is that the many challenges you face are good for you. They force you to grow. Without challenges, there is no growth. With no growth, there is stagnation. Learning and growth are lifelong processes. If you work your recovery well, you will always be becoming, changing, and growing for the rest of your life. Challenge is what makes life rich and meaningful. Challenge is what makes growth possible.

Think for a moment if you had no challenges. Nothing to nurture, nothing to do. Nothing to stimulate you. Without challenge, your life would be empty and boring. To have the rewards of achievement without the effort of challenges would make those rewards meaningless. It is in the overcoming of challenges that you will experience the most meaning and rewards.

Do not avoid the challenges ahead. Face them and embrace them. Make challenge your friend, for it is the path to growth. Challenge can be frustrating. Make it easier for yourself by breaking down your challenges into small steps. Then you can work on your challenges one small step at a time. This will keep you from becoming too overwhelmed.

Ask for help in meeting your challenges. If you are having cravings, call someone to talk them out. If you need to get to a meeting, ask someone for a ride. If you are unsure what to do, talk out your dilemma with as many experienced and wise people as possible. You can also look within and ask for help from your Higher Power, if you have one, or from the inner source of wisdom that lies within you.

65. No one recovers alone. Emotional support is crucial to recovery.

Just as no one lives a healthy life alone, so it is true that no one recovers alone. You will need support to recover. You may think that you need to be strong and do recovery work all on your own; however, all of us need to know when to ask for help—it's part of being independent. Develop your inner strength to the point where you are secure in reaching out for help.

We all need a power greater than ourselves to get by. This is a paradox, because you do want to take complete accountability for your life. Your success in your recovery is up to you. At the same time, it is up to you to ask for help when you need it. You cannot do this all by yourself. You need guidance, assistance, and support. We all need each other to get by.

Take this book for example. It is one of your companions to support and guide you on your journey of recovery. Hopefully there will be other books, videos, and podcasts that will also help you.

When you are hurt, angry, afraid, and lonely, you will need people to talk to. Talking out life's pains and difficulties with others will help you to feel better. Find safe, wise, and supportive people who listen well without giving too much advice. A good friend will validate you, help you to put things into perspective, and help you to feel better. They might share their own experience so that you feel less alone.

Although you always have the option to journal about your cravings or meditatively be with your addictive urges until they pass, you should also have five to ten recovery support people whom you can call when you have cravings. Use these supports to talk out your craving as I discussed in a previous lesson. Go to recovery meetings and get the names and phone numbers of five to ten people with three or more years of recovery. Then call these recovery supports on a regular basis to check in and get current.

You cannot know the complete truth of things on your own. We all have blind spots. Your friends and supports will have insights and perspectives on your difficulties that you do not. Others can help you to creatively brainstorm solutions to problems. It is good to trust and rely on your own experience, but always pass it by someone wise so that you do not fall into self-delusion. It is said that addiction is cunning and baffling. Our capacity to rationalize our behaviors and delude ourselves is astounding. This is why you need the kind and honest feedback of others to help you maintain clarity.

The opposite of addiction is connection with our fellow humans. Remember that recovery entails not only accessing a power greater than yourself, but also living for something greater than yourself. You want to expand your identity through your loving connections to others. Then you won't feel so alone. Keep in mind that you need support and validation, just like everyone else.

You have many difficult times ahead of you. You are going to need the support of those who care about you to endure and prevail. You may experience flare-ups of your addiction. You will fall and feel like giving up. Have the humility and strength to ask for help to get up and go on.

66. There is healing to be found in mutual help meetings.

We all benefit from the support, inspiration, guidance, and accountability that recovery support groups and recovery mentors can provide us. We find these people at mutual help meetings. In addition to helping us meet recovery mentors and other supports, mutual help meetings provide several other benefits:

- Group members provide support and validation. They reduce shame and provide solidarity in the struggle with addiction.

- Meetings help us remember we have an illness that for many requires lifelong management. They help keep the memory fresh and protect us against the disease of forgetfulness.

- Meetings offer recovery wisdom and guidance. This includes advice on how to manage stress, triggers, cravings, and other life challenges. They help us to develop more positive ways of coping.

- Group members offer hope and inspiration. If they can create good lives from the wreckage of their addictions, we can too.

- Meetings provide the opportunity to develop a sense of belonging, which counters loneliness, isolation, and alienation.

- Meetings provide the opportunity for the fulfillment of helping others through service work.

The twelve-step meeting concept was originally developed by Alcoholics Anonymous; the steps are a set of guiding principles outlining a course of action for recovery. Twelve-step meetings come in all shapes and sizes. There are speaker-discussion meetings, women's meetings, LGBT-friendly meetings, and many others. The best strategy for trying a twelve-step meeting is to go to ten or more different meetings to find a few that fit best for you. You can then focus on the style of meeting that best coincides with your comfort level.

Twelve-step fellowships emphasize gaining power over addiction by surrendering to a Higher Power to help with sobriety. Although many peoples' Higher Power is God, a Higher Power may be anything outside of you that helps keep you sober. It could be the group, your mentor, your therapist, your family or friends, your pet, or Nature. The proven efficacy of this approach confirms the simple truth that most people, especially those with severe addiction, cannot achieve recovery alone without the help of something greater than themselves. We all need help to get by.

Narcotics Anonymous (NA) is a twelve-step fellowship. It is the most well-known mutual help meeting for those recovering from addiction to narcotics and other substances. There are many mutual help meetings that can help you recover. They include:

- Narcotics Anonymous (NA): www.na.org
- Women for Sobriety (WFS): www.womenforsobriety.org
- SMART Recovery: www.smartrecovery.org
- Secular Organizations for Sobriety (SOS): www.sossobriety.org
- LifeRing: www.lifering.org
- Refuge Recovery: www.refugerecovery.org
- Celebrate Recovery: www.celebraterecovery.com

In any of the twelve-step meetings, you may hear references to God as a higher power. If you are agnostic or atheist, don't let this stop you from attending meetings. Everyone—including you—needs a power greater than themselves both to recover and to live life well. Instead of "Higher Power," you may wish to think of a "Greater Power." This could be the members of the group, your recovery mentor, your therapist, your medication, this book or other recovery literature, Nature, your pet, or your family and friends.

You don't have to agree with other people's views to benefit from their support. The key with all mutual help meetings is to exercise tolerance, live and let live, and take what's best for you while leaving behind ideas or concepts that don't appeal to you. In other words: Chew the meat and spit out the bones. Everyone's recovery path is unique to them.

Meetings are a tool you will need to learn to use skillfully. Follow these guidelines:

- Go early and stay late in order to get to know people.

- Stay away from the smokers. Associate with members who have renounced all addicting.

- Listen carefully. Make it a goal at each meeting to take away one useful life lesson.

- Identify with other people, but don't compare yourself to others.

- Socialize with those who have several years of stable, complete sobriety. People who are young and fragile in their recovery can jeopardize your recovery.

Go to available meetings in your area. Try them all on for size. Meetings vary in format, in the people attending, and in the "vibe" in the meeting. You want to know about all your meeting options. After you have attended different meetings several times in your area, you can decide which meetings are best for you. Then attend these few meetings regularly so that you develop consistent, stable, meaningful relationships with the other attendees.

Make it a priority to go to meetings. Do not let life get in the way unless you have a true emergency. You must put your recovery first to make it last. Too many people find themselves readdicting when they stop going to meetings.

Online Support Groups

In the Rooms: www.intherooms.org

Addiction Recovery Guide: addictionrecoveryguide.org

Addiction Survivors: addictionsurvivors.org

NA Chatroom: nachatroom.org

Soberistas: soberistas.com

Support Groups: supportgroups.com. This site covers a wide range of issues including: addiction, depression, anxiety, and suicide.

12 Step Forums: 12stepforums.net

Online forums provide convenience, anonymity, and safety. They are limited, however, because they don't allow you to develop relationships in person.

If you are feeling anxious about attending meetings, just go and listen for a while. You don't have to talk in the first few meetings. Talk when you are comfortable. Be patient with yourself. Give yourself time to become comfortable in a group. Your anxiety will gradually recede as your brain learns that you are safe.

If you are new to recovery, it is a good idea to go to one or more meetings a day. After several years of recovery, when your life is stable and everything is going well, you may be able to reduce the frequency of meetings. This usually takes about three to five years for most people. Many people go to a meeting a week for the rest of their lives in order to "keep the memory fresh." Meetings help keep complacency at bay.

Twelve-step fellowships are not religious organizations. Despite this, some people don't like either the spiritual overtones of the twelve-steps or the concept of surrender. For these people, other meeting options exist:

Women for Sobriety meetings employ thirteen principles to empower women in their recovery.

SMART Recovery focuses on support and self-empowerment in managing cravings by examining the "ABCs" of behavior: antecedents, behaviors, and consequences. Members practice thinking through cravings to the end consequences of acting versus not acting on them as a way of getting unhooked. Secular Organizations for Sobriety and LifeRing both allow for people to come together to discuss their lives. Members give and receive support without the spiritual overtones of the twelve-step fellowships.

Refuge Recovery is a Buddhist-based movement that emphasizes meditation and mindfulness as a pathway to freedom from cravings and compulsions. Members support each other in their practice to develop the capacity to sit with urges without needing to act on them.

Celebrate Recovery is a Christian-based recovery program that also leverages sharing and support of members around a common religion. Other religions offer similar recovery support meetings of their own.

No matter your preference or background, there is a mutual help program that can help you through these difficult times and deal with the hardships of addiction as they present themselves.

Meetings allow you to obtain recovery supports. They allow you to learn from the wisdom and experience of others. They inspire you when you see how others have prevailed in the face of their addiction. They also promote self-examination through self-expression. In short, meetings provide support and help you grow.

67. Recovery mentors or coaches can offer more than just support.

A recovery mentor serves as a support and guide during your healing and transformation. This person could be a sponsor from one of the twelve-step fellowships or from one of the many other mutual help organizations. He or she may just be someone who you like, respect, or admire, who has achieved several years of recovery. Or, you may wish to consider hiring a professional recovery coach; these are trained coaches, who can help you make life decisions.

At first, you may feel a resistance to having a mentor. You may find yourself coming up with various reasons not to have a mentor. For example, it may feel too scary or embarrassing to reveal yourself to another person. You may feel you don't need a mentor, that you can do recovery on your own. You may worry about someone saying "No," that they don't wish to be your mentor when you ask them. Don't worry about them saying no. If they do say no, it may be because they simply do not have the time or energy to help you. That is not about you. Don't take it personally.

Twelve-Step Programs

The "twelve-steps" are the guiding principles of many support groups; the steps were originally established by Alcoholics Anonymous. Twelve-step programs involve the following:

- Admitting that one cannot control one's addiction or compulsion
- Recognizing a greater power that can give strength
- Examining past errors with the help of a sponsor (experienced member)
- Making amends for these errors
- Learning to live a new life with a new code of behavior
- Helping others who suffer from the same addictions or compulsions

---

It does take humility and courage to ask someone to be your mentor—you're risking being open and transparent with them. But remember: No one is too good to not benefit from having a mentor, and no one is too bad to be unworthy of a mentor. You can supercharge your recovery by working with a recovery mentor. You deserve the best recovery possible.

Don't worry about burdening another person with your problems. The person who benefits the most from a mentor-mentee relationship is the mentor. You are giving someone a gift when you provide them the opportunity to mentor you.

An ideal recovery mentor has five years or more of sobriety, free from all addictive substances and behaviors, including smoking. They have renounced numbing pain with addictive pleasure.

The ideal recovery mentor is someone who is generally of the same gender as you. It should be someone who is older and wiser, who serves as a parental or older-sibling figure. When you listen to them, you should have a feeling of appreciation—a feeling of "I want what they have."

An ideal recovery mentor is tough, kind, and wise. They are tough in that they hold you accountable and call you on your dishonesty, your self-deception, and on any unwise or unskillful choices you make. They are kind, in that they are compassionate and never judge you as a person—they judge only the choices you make. They are wise in that they share from their own personal experience what they have learned that works.

Use your recovery mentor as a sounding board and an accountability figure. "Get current" with them daily, if possible. "Getting current" means telling them everything that is happening in your life, and everything you are thinking, feeling, and doing. Be completely transparent and honest. Do not withhold embarrassing material. Don't let shame or self-will cause you to keep secrets. It is said, "We are as sick as our secrets." Stay healthy by withholding nothing from your mentor. Tell the whole truth of things. Then process the truth. This will allow you to reset emotionally, deepen your understanding of yourself and others, and learn how to live a joyful life in recovery.

Take care to keep proper boundaries in your relationship with your recovery mentor. Recovery mentors are not friends or family members. Friends and family members are too emotionally involved with you to serve as objective sounding boards.

Picking the right recovery mentor can be challenging. One approach is to ask someone to be your temporary mentor while you continue to look for the right person. This provides you with support and guidance right away.

Keep in mind that things may not always work out with your recovery mentor. If you feel the relationship is unhelpful, you can always find another mentor, and thank your old mentor for their help.

68. Your family and loved ones can help you.

When your loved ones nag you, plead with you, threaten you, or abandon you, it only makes things worse. On the other hand, they also don't help you when they give you money for your addiction or enable you in other ways, even though that feels good to you. They may not understand addiction. They may find your behavior baffling, crazy-making, frustrating, and hurtful. If they can get some clarity about addiction, they will have more compassion and understanding. If they can get some guidance as to how to best help you, everyone will benefit.

There are four basic principles your loved ones can practice to help you in your recovery.

- They should reward you with their time, support, and praise when you are engaging in good recovery behaviors.

- They should withdraw their rewards when you are engaging in your addiction. This might include any material supports, such as a place to live.

- They should engage in kind, positive, supportive communication with you, even when you are addicting or are otherwise hurtful or destructive. Rather than saying, "You are a worthless loser," they might say, "When you addict and lie to me, it breaks my trust in you and leaves me feeling scared for you and frustrated with your behavior."

- They should not shield you from the natural negative consequences of your addiction and your addictive behaviors. If you spend all your rent money on drugs, for example, they should not help you with your rent. You need to feel the pain of your addiction, combined with hope, in order to wake up and choose recovery. As I talked about before, pain is your friend. When your loved ones shield you from the pain of addicting, they unwittingly perpetuate the addiction.

There are other things your loved ones should not do. They should not interact with you when you are drug-affected. They should also not emotionally abandon you if it is within their capacity to do so. Being in relationship with someone who is addicting is difficult and often very painful. It may take great emotional stamina for your loved ones to stay engaged with you.

Hopefully, your loved ones will provide you with unconditional love and emotional support. They may also need to provide you with the minimum of life-sustaining material support if it is a matter of life and death. Hopefully they will also help you to obtain treatment if you need help with this.

Your loved ones can also help you by having hope for you, believing in you, and expecting that you can recover. They can expect that you can care for yourself with the help of others, support yourself, and lead a life of love and integrity. They serve you best by having high but realistic expectations of you.

There are two good books your family and loved ones should read to help you recover. One is *Get Your Loved One Sober* by Meyers and Wolfe. The other is *Beyond Addiction* by Foote and Wilkens. Encourage your family members to buy and read these books. They will teach your loved ones how to love you skillfully in order to promote your recovery.

69. Your spirituality will help you with recovery.

It is said that addiction is a medical illness with a spiritual solution. What does that mean?

First of all, you may or may not consider yourself to be a spiritual person. The fact is, however, that everyone, even atheists, have spirituality, because spirituality is part of being human.

So let's start by first defining spirituality, then we can talk about how spirituality promotes recovery. I like to think of spirituality as a healthy relationship with Reality. When we are healthy spiritually, we feel a sense of being harmoniously connected to and a part of a greater, loving Reality. We feel we are a part of something good and greater than ourselves. We sense that the Universe is rigged in our favor. This experience of connectedness or unity generates feelings of love. Your spirituality creates feelings of reverence and respect for the One Life of which you are a part.

When you are spiritually healthy, you experience the truth that your life and all of Life is an incredible, miraculous, mystery worthy of your utmost reverence. You see the extraordinary in the ordinary. Life, including your life and the lives of others, is sacred, meaning it is of immeasurable value.

In addition to love, your spirituality also inspires feelings of wonder, awe, gratitude, humility, and acceptance. When you are spiritually healthy, you are right with Reality, including the inevitable pain of life. You live life out of love rather than being ruled by fear.

We cultivate our spirituality through stillness practices such as yoga, prayer, and meditation. These practices promote presence and connection before thought so that we can experience the bare truth of existence. We also cultivate our spirituality through living a reflective, thoughtful life.

So what does spirituality have to do with recovery? Here is the answer: addiction arises out of pain, and spirituality is the ultimate pain management solution. Your spirituality protects you from the pain that drives addiction and inspires you to act with love in everything that you say and do.

Think about it this way: If you truly felt that you, your life, and all of Life were sacred—if you felt a deep reverence for your life and the lives of others—would you do anything to harm yourself or others, even if you felt strong urges to do so?

The answer is "No." You would never do anything to harm yourself, including addicting. If you were out of control with addiction, you would humbly empower yourself by asking for help.

Since you know addicting is harmful, your spirituality protects you from acting on urges to addict out of your deep reverence for Life, including your life. Since your spirituality connects you to something greater than you, you tap into that "something more" to soothe and sustain you, whether it be the stillness of nature, the support of a friend, your pet, or the sense of an intelligent, loving force that some people experience as their "Higher Power." You can also think of this as a "Greater Power" because it is a force greater than you.

Your spirituality puts your pain in its proper perspective. Your reverence for Reality inspires an acceptance of this moment just as it is. Everything is perfectly imperfect, exactly as it must and can only be. Pain is a necessary part of Life. Our job is to resolve pain with love—either soothing ourselves or accepting pain we cannot relieve. With your healthy spirituality, you develop the capacity to experience peace in the midst of the storms of life, including the storm of addiction. This is why you should gently practice cultivating your spirituality every day. Your spirituality will serve you well in your recovery.

Spiritual people experience love in their relationships. They experience a sense of connectedness or oneness with others and with the whole of Reality. They experience an altruistic desire to help others. They act from their "Higher Self" rather than from their "Ego Self," which is concerned only with their own safety, comfort, and survival. They engage in spiritual practices like prayer and meditation. They live contemplative and reflective lives.

The experience of oneness and stillness produced by spiritual practices promotes a sense of the Sacred, and of awe and wonder. The practice of presence promotes perspective; you see that who you truly are is the deep, formless Awareness in which thoughts, feelings, and sensations arise. You see that you are not your thoughts, feelings, and sensations. This awakening leads to insight and wisdom into the true nature of things. When you are living from still presence, what I call "stillness in motion," the urges of the ego lose some of their power. You will find yourself less compelled to addict when cravings arise.

Your spirituality will help you to see that life is sacred and good. You will see that you exist to nurture and savor Life, including your own. You will see that Life is about Life, and your calling is to serve Life. Your spirituality will give you a deep sense of purpose and meaning, because you will experience yourself as being part of something greater than you that sustains you. Out of gratitude and reverence, you will feel the calling to serve with love.

Therefore, your spirituality will motivate you to live and act with love. As you cultivate your spirituality, you will find yourself developing several positive character traits, including self-awareness, love, altruism, peace, generosity, and contentment. You will be more compassionate and forgiving, both to yourself and to others.

When you live out of love, you experience the joy and fulfillment of love. This joy helps to protect you from cravings—life is just too good to give it all up for a drug. As you put love out into the world, love comes back to you to support and sustain you through difficult times. When you have an abiding sense of a loving and intelligent Reality that generously resonates with your love, you will develop a sense of peace and faith that all is well beneath the surface ripples of life's dramas and distresses. The fruits of spirituality—peace, faith, and love—will protect you from readdicting.

70. Spiritual practices promote recovery.

We know from the literature and from personal experience that spiritual practices promote recovery. Meditation, mindfulness, and prayer provide relief from suffering. They help repair compromised self-regulation caused by addiction and trauma. Several studies have shown meditation to be beneficial to recovery. In one study, time spent in meditation was a significant predictor of decreases in substance use. A recent study showed a zero percent return to drinking in three months with twice-daily transcendental meditation.

Studies have shown that meditation may promote recovery by reducing stress, depression, anxiety, and pain. Since pain fuels cravings to addict, the pain-reducing benefits of meditation appear to protect you.

A recent study showed that practicing yoga also reduced readdiction, perhaps by reducing stress. Spiritual practices promote the experience of unity or oneness. As I discussed in a previous lesson, this enhances your drive to live for something greater than yourself. Being part of something greater than yourself gives you purpose and meaning. We know that a higher sense of purpose and meaning will also protect you from readdicting.

Although meditation may sound complex, it is really a very simple practice. When you meditate, you pay attention to what is going on right now. Most people start meditation by focusing on their breath. You gently and repeatedly pull Awareness out of its immersion in thought so that Awareness can experience the Now.

After focusing on your breathing, you might also notice what you see, what you feel in your body, and what you hear. You might then notice your thoughts and feelings, trying not to get lost in them. When you are beginning meditation, you are probably best off returning your attention over and over again back to your breathing when you notice that your mind has wandered.

One form of meditation that I particularly like is to memorize and quietly recite a spiritual passage. A good one, for example, is a prayer by St. Francis of Assisi:

Lord, make me an instrument of thy peace.
Where there is hatred, let me sow love;
Where there is injury, pardon;
Where there is doubt, faith;
Where there is despair, hope;
Where there is darkness, light;
Where there is sadness, joy.

O divine Master, grant that I might not so much seek
To be consoled as to console,
To be understood as to understand,
To be loved as to love.
For it is in giving that we receive,
It is in pardoning that we are pardoned,
It is in dying to self that we are born to eternal life.

Repeat this prayer slowly, focusing on the meaning of the words. When your mind wanders, start back at the beginning. Say it over and over. You can meditate either sitting still or while engaging in a repetitive task such as walking, running, chanting, or counting beads.

Mindfulness is meditation in motion. It is the practice of noticing what is going on right now, with an attitude of friendly, nonjudgmental appreciation of all experience, whether painful or pleasurable. You develop the sense of being still, even while moving. This is the practice of presence. When you are present, you are very aware of compulsions and cravings to addict. When you are present, you are tapped into the stillness that exists beneath all experience. This stillness will help you in your recovery. When you are still, you will find you are less hooked by cravings. The compulsive quality of cravings will recede. You will feel more grounded and centered. You will be better able to maintain the "big picture" of things—that you are a sacred being having a temporary experience of cravings.

Your stillness will help you to pause and process your experience, as you consider the question, "What would love do?" Stillness thus gives you the freedom to do the next right thing, whether it be to call someone to talk out your cravings or to do what this moment calls for.

Another spiritual practice is contemplation. In stillness, you ask a question of yourself, over and over, such as, "What is the loving thing to do in this situation?" You ask, and then listen for the answer, in stillness and silence.

In prayer, you can either pray with words, or engage in silent, contemplative prayer. The intent of prayer is generally to connect with a transcendent life force, which some call God. You might also pray if you're an atheist. In this case your communication is with your unconscious inner source of wisdom or with someone that you completely trust. Your intent should be to express yourself completely, with complete honesty and transparency, while opening your heart to all that you feel.

There are three types of prayer: "Help," "Thanks," and "Wow." When asking for help, don't ask for a particular outcome. Ask for understanding, strength, faith, hope, guidance, peace, insight, wisdom, and acceptance. When you say, "Thanks," you express gratitude for the gift of your life and for your many blessings. When you say, "Wow," you experience the wonder, the sacredness, and the awe of existence.

With word prayers, focus on the meaning of the words. Go beyond the words to experience the truth to which they point. In contemplative prayer, you ask a question or silently repeat a word or phrase. A question might be, "What does Life need from me?" Then listen carefully for the silent answer. As Father Thomas Keating, a Catholic monk said, "God speaks to us in silence. Everything else is a bad translation." In contemplation, you ask. When you go into the stillness of contemplative prayer, you listen for the answers. In repeating a mantra, such as "one" or "surrender," you focus on the meaning of the word and then listen for the wordless response.

The process of prayer is mysterious. Your intentional efforts combined with allowance create the conditions for insight and transformation to occur. Nonreligious contemplation is very similar to contemplative prayer, with the difference being that you are not imagining an answer from a higher being. As in all contemplation, you focus your attention on an important concern, such as, "What would make my life more meaningful?" You ask, and then listen, in stillness and silence, for the answer to come.

In all contemplation, return your awareness over and over again back to the one thought that is your question. You are like the person before dawn, sitting in the darkness, waiting for the sun to rise. The answers may come gradually, a piece at a time, in many forms, over a lifetime. Often, the answers start out as general principles that become more detailed and specific over time. For many, the answers change over time with the accumulation of knowledge, experience, awareness, and wisdom.

Be steady, patient, persistent, and consistent in your spiritual practice. Never let life get in the way of your spiritual practice. Schedule it at the beginning of each day with a time for reflection at the end of each day. Give it time. Make a steady, gentle effort. In doing so, you will progress. You will experience setbacks and plateaus. Do not give up. Consistent, gentle, steady effort will eventually yield freedom from addiction, relief from suffering, and enhanced wisdom, joy, and vitality.

71. Recovery requires thoughtfulness and caution.

You know that because of your addiction you cannot completely trust your mind. In particular, you cannot always trust the impulses that arise from your brain's drive-reward system. Because of your addiction, your drive-reward system is programmed to drive you to addict to feel better now. It is not taking into account messages from your brain's frontal lobes telling it that addicting will result in disastrous consequences. This is the essence of the illness of addiction.

Because you suffer from addiction, you will need to practice thoughtfulness and caution. Thoughtfulness entails stopping when you have an urge to do something to carefully think through the consequences. Do this by passing all your thoughts by a recovery support. Especially in early recovery, you don't want to do anything of consequence before you have passed it by your recovery mentor or another recovery support. If you are thinking of calling an old friend who may still be addicting, for example, talk it through with your recovery support. Don't take any actions of consequence until you have thought them through by talking them out. This is part of your daily practice of getting current. Knowing you have a vulnerability in decision making, become humble and get help from people you trust. Don't take action until you have carefully considered all your options and have weighed the pros and cons of each option. You will know what is best for you when you know what is best for you. Clarity will come after a process of careful deliberation.

Knowing you have vulnerability, you also need to be cautious. You need to avoid unnecessary risks. It there is a party you'd like to go to where there might be drugs, caution would counsel you to not go. If you don't want to slip, you need to avoid slippery situations.

Life can be dangerous. You need to look both ways before crossing the street. You also need to be cautious in your dealings with others. Not everyone is highly evolved in their capacity to love. Many people will hurt you or exploit you if you allow them to. You need to take care to protect yourself from unnecessary harm. A good rule of thumb is to trust people to do only what they feel is in their best interest.

Be very cautious in dealing with people in early recovery. Remember that in many ways they are just like you. Their vulnerability to readdicting can trigger your readdicting. A cautious rule that will serve you well is to not socialize with anyone with less than three years of solid recovery. This will mean you will need to say good-bye to your friends who are addicting or who are in early recovery. Although this can be painful, it is the cautious thing to do.

Your life is precious. You have a lot on the line with a lot to lose. There are likely many people who are impacted by the choices you make. You suffer from an illness that impairs judgment. For all these reasons, commit yourself to living a thoughtful, cautious life. Trust the counsel of the wise and loving people who surround you. Avoid all unnecessary risks. Take your time to process things with others until you are quite clear on the best course of action.

72. Serving others will help you.

A friend of mine shared the following story with me:

An Indian businessman, dripping with gold and diamonds, came one day to visit Mother Teresa, the nun known worldwide for her acts of kindness, fell at her feet, and proclaimed, "Oh God, you are the holiest of the Holy! You are the super-holy one! You have given up everything! I cannot even give up one samosa for breakfast! Not one single piece of bread for lunch can I give up!"

Mother Teresa started to laugh so hard her attendant nuns grew scared. Mother Teresa was in her middle 80s and frail from two recent heart attacks. Eventually, she stopped laughing and, wiping her eyes with one hand, she leaned and said softly, "So you say I have given up everything?"

The businessman nodded enthusiastically.

Mother Teresa smiled. "Oh, my dear man," she said, "you are so wrong. It isn't I who have given up everything. It is you. You have given up the supreme, sacred joy of life, the source of all lasting happiness, the joy of giving your life away to other beings, to serve the Divine in them with compassion. It is you who has given up everything!"

To the Indian businessman's total bewilderment, Mother Teresa got down on her knees and bowed to him.

Flinging up his hands, he ran out of the room.

Much of your unhappiness, addiction, and depression spring from our "Big Me" culture of self-preoccupation with achievement, wealth, and compulsive consumption, spurred by the relentless media messages telling you what you need to buy and what you need to be to be happy. In this way, our culture is diseased. We are one of the wealthiest nations on earth, yet many live joyless, addiction-ridden lives.

We have lost touch with the timeless wisdom of compassionate service, the gift of joy we give ourselves when we give to others. The Buddhist mystic Shantideva spoke to this:

All the joy the world contains
Has come through wishing happiness for others;
All the misery the world contains
Has come through wanting pleasure for oneself.

We lose joy and happiness when we grasp for them. Reflect on the people you know. Reflect on the times when you have felt truly happy and fulfilled. You will notice that you and others experience the greatest joy when you are nurturing Life. This is why devoting yourself to the well-being of others is so critical to your own well-being.

If you wish for happiness, joy, and fulfillment, make a commitment, on purpose, to a daily, intentional practice of service to others. Ask yourself, "What does the world ask of me?" Look and listen for your higher purpose to be revealed. If something is blocking you, such as resentments, negativity, victim thinking, compulsive consumerism, self-preoccupation, or self-gratification, mindfully note these unskillful habits of mind and let them go. This will clear the way for your Higher Self to develop. As you allow yourself to become a channel of love, the experience of dissatisfaction and lack will dissolve.

Giving is a gift you give yourself. When you love others, you experience the fulfillment of loving. You feel lovable through loving. Loving makes you whole. Protect your recovery by serving others. It will be you who benefits the most.

73. Recovery is a lifelong practice.

Recovery is not something you do until you are sober and then stop. Becoming sober is just the beginning of a life-long practice. You can stop working on your recovery when you die, but not before then.

Recovery is a process of continuous growth and transformation. It is not an event. It is a journey, not a destination. Recovery is a practice. Like any practice, it requires consistency and repetition, day after day after day. Recovery does not get a day off. Keep in mind that if you are not moving away from your addiction in recovery, you may well be moving toward it.

The biggest room in life is the room for improvement. What is wonderful about recovery is that, through your daily practice of recovery, you will experience the incredible rewards of continuous growth and transformation. You will hit plateaus, to be sure. But with persistence and consistency, you will attain more and more wisdom, clarity, skill, joy, and fulfillment.

Remember that it is in your nature to addictively numb pain with pleasure. You will need to steadily swim against the stream of this "brain desire" for the rest of your life. Recovery is like turning the crank on a light generator. When you stop turning the crank, the light goes out.

I can't tell you how many times I've admitted patients to detox because they stopped working on their recovery. They thought they were beyond their addiction. They let life get in the way of their recovery practices. They developed complacency. They stopped swimming against the stream of their addiction, and the stream of their addiction swept them back into addicting.

Guard yourself against complacency. When you don't feel you need to work on your recovery, that is the time you need to work your recovery the most.

Remember that for many people addiction does not ever go away. It only goes into remission. You will need to engage in a lifelong practice of recovery to prevent flare-ups of addicting. This means taking good care of yourself, managing stress skillfully, keeping up with a regular spiritual practice, getting current with one or more people daily, and living a life of love from your Higher Self.

All of these activities require intentional effort and practice. In recovery, you live your life intentionally, on purpose. When you lose your commitment and discipline, you will know that you are off track.

After a while, you will taste the fruits of recovery and realize for yourself how incredibly fulfilling recovery can be. Experiencing the rewards of recovery will hopefully inspire you to keep on keeping on with your recovery work. Make a promise to yourself that you will develop and maintain your recovery habits for the rest of your life. It is through the process of continuous growth and renewal that you will optimize your vitality and keep addiction at bay.

PART V
What You Need to Know about Healing

74. Seek healing from past trauma and neglect.

After you stop addicting, you will need to turn your efforts toward healing your emotional trauma, as well as any neglect you might have suffered growing up. The pain of trauma and neglect drive addicting to numb that pain. If you do not address this pain, you will be more vulnerable to readdicting.

Trauma and neglect damage your capacity to feel safe, secure, and trusting. Neglect and trauma leave victims with a terrible feeling of being empty, broken, and unlovable. Trauma and neglect damage the emotional-relational part of the brain that gives you your sense of self and allows for you to safely engage in loving and being loved.

One of the key riddles of life that you will need to solve is how to be both independent and dependent on others at the same time. What this means is that we are separate people responsible for our own lives, but at the same time we need each other to get by. Knowing when to rely on others will allow you to realize self-fulfillment as well as the fulfillment of loving and being loved. Trauma and neglect damage the ability to solve this riddle.

If you have suffered from trauma and neglect, you have probably endured many negative emotions, including:

- Helplessness and powerlessness
- Alienation
- Emptiness
- Hurt

- Anger
- Bitterness
- Resentment
- Irritability
- Suspiciousness
- Self-hatred
- Hatred of others
- Sadness and grief
- Betrayal
- Desire for revenge

All of these negative emotional states need healing and resolution, because they will fuel cravings to numb your pain, which will fuel readdicting.

To realize joy in your recovery, you will need to feel good about yourself, good about others, and good about life. You will need to feel empowered, safe, and secure. You will need to know how to protect yourself from harm, how to set limits with others, and how to skillfully trust others in ways they can be trusted. These are all emotional and relational capacities that are damaged by trauma and neglect. This is why the second phase of recovery entails emotional and relational rehabilitation.

Find a good therapist who is skilled both in treating addictions and in treating trauma and neglect. Your therapist will coach you through the stages of healing from trauma:

- Establishing safety and stabilizing painful emotions
- Processing and mourning trauma and neglect
- Cultivating a wise and compassionate perspective on what you have endured
- Reconnecting safely and skillfully with others and with your life
- Developing a trauma-informed spirituality. This means restoring a sense of the Universe as being a good and loving place despite the reality of evil and trauma.

If you have difficulties safely loving and being loved, join a long-term process psychotherapy group, where you can safely learn how to be respectfully authentic with others. How you address your trauma and neglect will determine the course of your life. Even though you can't change what happened to you, you can choose to heal, and in doing so, change your future.

Most people who have healed from trauma and neglect say they grew spiritually in ways they might not have grown if it were not for their trauma. They developed wisdom, compassion, and the capacity to forgive others, themselves, and Life Itself. I pray that through healing from your trauma that you will emerge from the fire of your trauma a shining star so that you can light the way for others who have suffered as you have.

75. Be accountable to yourself. Move from victim to survivor.

You, and you alone, are responsible for your success in life and for your recovery. It may not seem fair, but it's the truth. You are not a victim. You are a survivor. It is up to you to ask for the help you need to heal and recover. You can succeed at life with the help, support, and guidance of others, but you need to take accountability for yourself. Living your life is your responsibility, no one else's.

Several life practices make up the practice of accountability.

First, you must take good care of yourself. It is your responsibility to care for yourself as if you were your own ideal parent. You need to nurture your well-being to optimize your vitality. You also need to take accountability for not harming yourself in any way.

Second, you should take accountability for savoring this precious gift of life. Practice grateful appreciation for the miraculous experience of consciousness. Life is to be lived in this moment.

Third, practice positivity. See the opportunity in every difficulty. It is in the overcoming of difficulties that you experience much of your happiness and fulfillment. As mentioned earlier, remember that pain is your friend, because it sternly informs you that you are somehow not right with Life.

Mindfully note negative judgments about yourself and others and gently release them with compassion both for yourself and others. Be kind, supportive, and giving to both yourself and others. With a positive perspective, you will respond positively to life's difficulties, resulting in positive outcomes.

Given where I was, this great new life seems like a miracle. I feel so lucky, but I also know that it was me who decided to get sober.

Liz, 44

Fourth, stop blaming others for your emotions or behaviors. You alone are responsible for how you respond to what life throws at you. You always have a choice. Take accountability for all your actions and reactions. It is up to you to choose to act with love and integrity from moment to moment.

Fifth, take accountability for managing your vulnerabilities. If you are vulnerable to being selfish, own this and renounce behaving selfishly. If you are vulnerable to being hurtful, renounce this and vow to do no harm. If you are vulnerable to being dishonest, renounce this and vow to be honest. If you are vulnerable to retreating from situations out of fear, renounce this and act with courage. Take accountability for countering your flaws with the practice of virtue for the rest of your life. With time, the practice of virtue will become habit, replacing old, destructive habits.

Sixth, take responsibility for living for a higher purpose. You are meant to live your life not only to savor Life, but also to nurture Life in ways that are unique to you. Look within. Listen to your soul. Look without. What calls to you from within? How does Life call to you? Take accountability for answering these calls.

Seventh, take accountability for overcoming your fears. This includes fears of failure, rejection, harm, or loss. Life requires courage. At times you will need to take risks to do what is right. If you struggle with fear, get help from a therapist.

Finally, take accountability for achieving your key life goals. Commit yourself to your success. Create a plan of action and act. Overcome the obstacles that arise. Persist and persevere. Never give up. Try, and keep on trying. Believe in yourself. Get the help, support, and guidance you need to succeed.

When you take accountability for your life, you empower yourself to succeed. Believe in yourself, and surround yourself with people who believe in you. You can and will have a happy and successful life when you decide to do so.

76. Practice loving yourself.

Authentic recovery from addiction is impossible when you hate yourself. Recovery is the practice of love, including love for yourself. As you stop addicting, you also need to stop hating yourself or hurting yourself in any way.

You are an amazing creation of the Universe. Hold yourself with reverence and gratitude, despite your many flaws, deficiencies, failures, mistakes, diseases, and disabilities. You are of infinite, immeasurable value. You are sacred. See this, and love yourself as if you were your own cherished child. Reverently and radically accept yourself just as you are, right here, right now. Healing starts with loving self-acceptance. See that you are both beautiful and imperfect, just like everyone else.

Appreciate your talents and achievements. Feel grateful for your gifts and proud for your achievements. Dissolve self-hatred. When negative, judgmental thoughts and emotions arise, mindfully note them. Lovingly thank them for arising in your consciousness. Then replace them with an opposite, more realistic, positive thought of valuing, appreciation, acceptance, and gratitude. Show yourself deep compassion for your suffering.

Renounce all addicting. It is simply not loving to destroy yourself through addiction. You cannot learn to resolve pain with love if you continue to numb it through addicting. Choose recovery, ask for help, and set yourself free.

Ensure your safety and secure your basic needs. Assert yourself and protect yourself. Set limits on others as needed. Remove yourself from destructive people, places, and things. Place yourself in a positive recovery environment.

As discussed, take accountability for your life. This is an act of self-love. Take ownership of your destructive behavior while maintaining compassion for yourself. Name, claim, and tame your vulnerabilities while appreciating your innate goodness. Set goals and go for them. Pursue your passions and dreams.

Surround yourself with loving people. You need loving connections with others to survive and thrive. In doing so, devote yourself to loving them. Practice honesty, care, humility, and respect. Affirm others. Be generous. Give of your time and attention. Love others without conditions or expectations. If the thought arises to do something kind for someone, do it. You will feel more lovable the more you love others. You will notice that in loving others, you fill your own emptiness.

Take good care of your body and brain. Eat right, get plenty of sleep, rest, and exercise regularly. Take time to rest, relax, play, and have fun. Simplify and balance your life; minimize your stress. Live with contentment. Work on your recovery every day to keep addiction at bay.

Get treatment for medical and mental illnesses and to heal from trauma. Your self-love is the fundamental act of recovery. Self-love also enables you to love others. With time, your practice of self-love and love for others will create a loving and self-rejuvenating resonance with Reality. You will shift from feeling un-whole to experiencing "imperfect wholeness." In the fullness of love, you will find yourself protected from readdicting.

77. Avoid hurtful relationships.

If you are like most people, you likely have some relationships that are harmful to you. Because pain feeds addiction, you will want to either end relationships with those who are harmful to you or modify your interactions so that you are not harmed. You will be fragile in your early recovery. Harm to you will harm your healing and growth. This is why you need to avoid hurtful relationships.

You may have relationships with others who also suffer from addiction. People possessed by addiction cannot be true friends. Since addiction makes the primary purpose in life to serve the addiction, victims of addiction cannot make you, or anyone else for that matter, their first priority. People who suffer from addiction are hurtful to you. What may look like friendship is in reality a relationship of convenience that revolves around addicting. Your addicting "friends" will want you to addict as well in order to normalize and support their addicting. Because of their disabled capacity to love, they will not be thinking of what is best for you. Lost in their addiction, they cannot generate the kind of consciousness that will support your recovery.

By letting go of shame, I've learned to be assertive. I'm trusting myself and my intuition. It's like learning to be humble and open to what others have to say and trusting yourself at the same time.

Ann, 47

You should end all relationships with anyone who is addicting. You can do so kindly, with compassion. But be firm. Tell them that because you are in recovery, you cannot be around people who use drugs, as they will trigger you to use. You can wish them well and tell them you would be happy to reconnect with them after they have had a few years of solid recovery themselves.

Take inventory of all your relationships. Who else in your life causes you harm? Who disregards your needs? Who invalidates you? Who is abusive to you? Who attempts to exploit you? Make a list. For each person, write out the ways they harm you or fail to love you. Clarify the reality of things. Have the courage to be very honest with yourself and those who love you.

Once you've made this list, reflect on each person on the list. Notice your feelings toward them. Especially notice feelings of attachment or dependence. You may say to yourself, "But I love them!" and think that enduring their harm is better than losing the relationship.

If you think someone will respond if you set limits with them and ask them to stop harming you, great! Assert yourself, kindly and firmly. We all need limits set on us from time to time to prevent us from consciously or unconsciously taking advantage of others. If your friend or loved one responds to your asserting yourself and stops harming you, then that is a relationship you may be able to salvage.

Some of your friends and loved ones may not respond to your assertiveness. They may continue to hurt you. When this happens, you need to either end the relationship or severely restrict it so that you are no longer harmed.

Ending or limiting harmful relationships can be painful because of your attachments to those who harm you. You may feel you deserve to be mistreated. You may feel it would be worse to be alone than to be with someone who harms you. I am here to tell you that you do not deserve to be harmed and that you are better off surrounding yourself with people who love you. Breaking attachments can be painful. You will need courage, clarity, resolve, and the support of those who love you. Just know that protecting yourself from harm by others is absolutely essential for your healing and recovery. Knowing this, do what you must to protect yourself from harm.

78. Understand the power in loving others.

If you suffer from addiction, it is true that at some level you likely hate yourself because of all the destructive things you have done to yourself and to others. If you're like the majority of people who suffer from addiction, on some level you may feel you are unlovable or unworthy.

If this is true for you, know that you are not alone. Most people who suffer from addiction feel broken, unworthy, unwhole, or unlovable.

The cure for this is love. If you feel unlovable, you can change this feeling by loving yourself and others. It is a simple truth that the way to feel lovable is to be loving. Love heals.

You will find that people will be more loving to you on the whole if you are a loving person. Actions have consequences. If you act with love, the law of karma will result in love coming back to you. You will create a virtuous cycle of loving resonance that will benefit everyone. The loving response of others to your loving will help you to feel more lovable.

It may seem that there is contradiction here, however. Loving others in order to receive something in return from them is not love—it is barter. You must love for love's sake alone and for no other reasons. For your love to be true, it must be without expectations.

But this is okay, because loving others feels good. It is good for you. When you do or say something that benefits another, that benefit is reward enough. You will find it spiritually rejuvenating.

Ideally, as you grow spiritually, you will reach a point where you do not feel the need for the love of everyone to sustain you. You will feel unconditionally lovable because of your practice of love. Then you will be truly free to love and to speak your truth without fear. This will be liberating. In the meantime, embrace the love of others to support and sustain you as you heal and grow.

The fulfillment of loving is far more rewarding than the gratification of painkillers. Loving others will reduce cravings for painkillers, because life will be too good to give up for a temporary opioid high and all the pain that follows.

It is in loving yourself and others that you heal your brokenness. It is through loving that you become whole. Start each day with an intention to love yourself and others in all you say and do. Look for opportunities throughout the day to benefit others. You will find this practice deeply rewarding, joyful, and healing.

79. Live your life with integrity.

Integrity means to be honest, ethical, and moral in your conduct. When you have integrity, you live according to a higher set of love-based moral principles such as honesty, mutuality, and collaboration. Not only will others know you are honest and ethical, but also you will know.

Integrity is about doing the next right thing from moment to moment regardless of urges to do otherwise. It is about acting with virtue. It is about doing what is best for everyone, including yourself. When you have integrity, what you think, say, and do are in harmony. You walk your talk. You are trustworthy. You are reliable.

You are part of the One Life that sustains you. It is a simple truth that, because of our interdependence, if you hurt others for selfish gain, you ultimately hurt yourself. This is why acting with integrity is good for you. If you put good out into the world, good comes back to you. If you put bad out into the world, that comes back to you as well.

When you act with integrity, you live for both yourself and for the One Life of which you are a part. You balance your concern for yourself with a concern for others. You refrain from acting with selfish disregard for others. You do not exploit others or manipulate others for your gain alone.

In your healing and recovery, you will need to practice meticulous honesty in all your affairs. This includes being honest with yourself. Someone else may not know you did something wrong, but you know.

The only time you might withhold the truth is when it would cause harm. If you are like most people, you have lied to manipulate others to give you something you wanted or to avoid painful consequences of your unskillful behavior. This will need to stop. You will need to take accountability for the consequences of your behavior. See that dishonesty separates you from others, causes guilt and shame, and ultimately harms you as much as it can harm others.

There will be times when you will be afraid of doing the next right thing. If you break an object, you may fear admitting it because you fear someone's angry reaction or that you might have to pay for the broken item. This is an example of where integrity calls upon you to own up to what you did despite your fear of the consequences.

To live with integrity is to live without regrets or remorse. Integrity enhances your self-esteem, because your actions are esteem-able. Acting with integrity reduces shame and fear. When you act with integrity, you don't have to look back over your shoulder, fearing some negative consequence of unjust behavior on your part. If you don't break the law, for example, you don't have to worry as much about getting arrested and put in prison. Integrity gives you peace of mind.

When you act with integrity, you commit to not causing harm. This includes not harming yourself by numbing pain with pleasure through addicting. Because of your integrity, you put love for yourself and others before destructive gratification.

Acting without integrity not only harms you in the long run, it also creates stress, which triggers cravings to addict. When you act with integrity, you not only enhance your well-being, you also protect your recovery.

80. Learn to be assertive and how to protect your emotional boundaries.

Assertiveness and boundaries are both necessary for love. Your recovery requires that you develop healthy relationships. Healthy relationships require that you be assertive and enforce personal boundaries.

Assertiveness means to take care of yourself with others by both asking for what you need from others and also asking for others to not do things that are harmful to you. At the same time, assertiveness includes respecting the needs, rights, feelings, and opinions of others. Thus you might ask someone not to yell at you or to clean up after themselves.

Boundaries are also necessary for love. You need to enforce boundaries with your loved ones in order to protect your privacy and your limits. Examples of setting boundaries include privacy when you use the restroom. Other examples might be asking a loved one to not read your journal or to respect your need for alone time. While we are all interdependent, we are also autonomous, or independent. We have separate selves. We all see things differently. We think differently. We don't all have the exact same beliefs, values, preferences, or opinions. Our boundaries help us realize our differentiation from one another out of respect for the fact that we are each separate human beings.

When you are assertive and enforce your boundaries, be clear, firm, and kind. Say what you mean, but don't say it in a mean way. One strategy is the "ABCD" formula: "When you do A, I feel B, I need to ask that you do C, or else I will do D." Here's an example. If someone does something upsetting, for example, let's say showing up late for dinner without letting you know, you might say, "When you are late for dinner, I feel upset. I need for you to be on time or call me to let me know you are running late, or I will eat dinner without you."

Boundaries and assertiveness are essential, because we all have egos—our personal sense of "I". Out of our needs for safety, comfort, and status, we are all vulnerable to selfishness. If you act like a doormat, even the greatest of saints will wipe their feet on you. You help others to be their best and to live out of love when you assert yourself and enforce your boundaries.

You may have difficulties asserting yourself or enforcing your boundaries out of fear of rejection or lack of self-regard. You may have learned that taking care of yourself is "selfish." If this is the case, know that asserting yourself is good for everyone and that it is both your right and your duty, as you are responsible for taking good care of yourself. You will need to get comfortable with others being upset with your setting limits and asking for what you need. Pleasing everyone at all costs is not good for you. Accept and love yourself, and relieve others of the obligation to accept and love you. If you act with love and integrity, you are okay, no matter what anyone else thinks.

81. Know that there is joy in loving Life.

If you pause for a moment to be still, you can see the obvious right in front of you: You are Life aware of Itself. You have been blessed with the extraordinary gift of self-aware consciousness. You will see that this eternal, ever-changing moment of Awareness is sacred. This is the plain truth of who you are. How incredible is it that Life has bestowed this gift upon you.

You can also see that you are part of a vast, interdependent, dynamic web of life that sustains you. Imagine if suddenly there were no life on this planet except for you? You would likely be dead in a matter of weeks. Life feeds on life, and life sustains life. If it were not for all the life that surrounds you, you would cease to be. This realization inspires a deep gratitude for the Life that sustains you. This gratitude, in turn, promotes your healing.

When you awaken to the truth that you are part of a larger Life force, you will notice that feelings of humble respect and reverence arise for the One Life of which you are a part. You will see that Life is about Life—Life is not about you except to the degree that you are a part of the web of Life. This is humbling. It puts things into their proper perspective. Life is lovingly about you, but it isn't *all* about you. There are much larger forces at play. When you truly see this, your reverence and humility will heal your hurts and resentments. In this way your love for Life will help you heal.

When seeds are cast upon the wind, some will land in fertile soil and thrive. Others will land among the rocks and die. We, too, have been cast about by the winds of fate. We were all dealt a more or less favorable hand of genetic cards when we were born. We were all subjected to traumas, trials, and tribulations. Yet there is also grace. There is grace that you are still alive despite all that you have been through. There is grace that you are able to read this book. There is grace that good treatments exist to help you heal. There is grace in the fact of Love. There is grace in the reality of the literally millions upon millions of people who have all contributed over hundreds of thousands of years to creating the conditions in which you now live. See this grace at play in your own life. No matter the trauma and hardships you have suffered, there is a loving life force available to help you heal. Seeing the reality of the grace of life will also help you to heal.

Life needs your love. As you love Life, you enhance the vitality of Life, and enhance Life's capacity to sustain and enhance your life. Seeing that you are part of this One Life, you see that loving Life is actually loving yourself indirectly. When you help heal the world, you heal yourself.

82. Connection with others is important to your recovery.

If you are like the vast majority of people suffering from addiction, you also suffer from a lack of loving connection. In fact, it was likely this lack of loving connection that, along with your genetics, drove you to addiction.

The opposite of addiction is connection. We all need each other to get by in life, as life is challenging. The problems and difficulties of life are many. They do not cease until the day we die. It is in the overcoming of these difficulties, with the help of others, that we realize fulfillment and happiness.

You will need the love, the wisdom, the support, and the guidance of those who love you to help you overcome life's difficulties, including the difficulty of your addiction. Since life entails pain, and pain triggers cravings, your connections will help you to deal with the pain of life and protect you from readdicting.

A pain shared is a pain halved. Two minds tending to a problem are better than one. Life is a team sport. Don't try to live it alone. You will benefit from the loving support and guidance of others.

I used to wake up every single day, feeling nonstop shame, disgust, and despair. But now, I've forgiven myself. I live my life every day to the fullest. If I could change the past, I would. But, I can't change it. So, I've just had to let it go and let the past be.

Howard, 26

None of us sees things perfectly clearly. We all have blind spots. We need the eyes of others to see what we cannot see. You will need the loving feedback of others to see yourself and your situation clearly.

Like everyone else, you have an ego. You are vulnerable to selfishness and the disregard of others. You will need loving connections with others to help you live out of love. You cannot love others if you do not have connections with them.

Without loving connections, you will continue to feel alienation. Separation, loneliness, and emptiness arise out of disconnection. All of these negative mind states prevent healing and promote addicting.

In your healing, you do not live for yourself alone. You live for others, for the One Life of which you are a part. You do this through the channel of your loving connections to others.

You have relationships that you have damaged by virtue of your addiction and other unskillful behaviors. For you to heal, you will need to heal these relationships by doing what you can to help others whom you have harmed to heal. This occurs through the process of making amends and restitution. Heal your relationships by making amends and restitution wherever possible. First, inquire. Seek to understand the harm you have caused. Then reflect back your understanding and express your authentic remorse for the harm you have caused. Then vow to never cause such harm again and follow through on your promise. Make restitution wherever possible. If you stole money, for example, pay it back.

A loving network of loving relationships will sustain you. Be very intentional about opening your heart to the people you can trust. Be open-hearted also in your giving of love to those around you. Your love will nourish and sustain your connections, which will then nourish and sustain your healing.

83. Learn to be humble.

Many people who suffer from addiction have a lack of self-love as well as a lack of love for others. This happens when they have had trauma and neglect. As a result, they are egomaniacs with inferiority complexes. If that is true for you, your healing will require humility.

Humility, being modest about yourself, starts with the practice of self-love. Humility allows you to experience yourself as simultaneously sacred and imperfect. You are neither grandiose nor inferior. You are "right-sized." You recognize both your strengths and your weaknesses. You see your accomplishments and your failings. You are realistic about yourself because you love yourself, just as you are.

Humility allows you to feel that you are special, but no more special than anyone else. This is the opposite of a sense of entitlement, in which you feel your needs and wishes are important and those of others are not. It is also a cure for narcissism because you see that your quest to be special is futile. Out of humility, you turn your efforts from attempts to be special to attempts to be helpful. This is far more rewarding.

When you are humble, you are grateful for your talents and gifts, not proud. Pride poisons humility, because it allows you to put yourself above others. In your practice of humility, be grateful for who you are, but not proud. Don't counter your lack of self-love by setting yourself above others. See that you are special, but no more special than anyone else.

Humility promotes self-forgiveness. If you are hard on yourself, see that you are because you grandiosely expect yourself to be perfect. Let go of this hidden grandiosity. Be humble. You are just another imperfect, beautiful person on the bus, just like everyone else. Humbly do your best, knowing that even doing your best will inevitably entail mistakes and failures.

Humility will relieve you of the need to be right all the time. This will open you up to the possibility of learning and growth. Your humility will make you teachable.

Your humility will endear you to others, for they will know that you value them just as much as you value yourself. They will feel that you care about their well-being, and not your self-aggrandizement. They will appreciate that when you are praised, you point out with gratitude those who helped you along the way. Rather than elevating yourself, you will spend more time elevating others.

Humility is good for you. Cultivate it by combining honest self-inquiry with loving self-acceptance of yourself, exactly as you are, with all your flaws and failings. See your miniscule but precious part in the big scheme of life. See that, just like everyone else, you are not perfect. Accept that you will make mistakes for the rest of your life. Your humble self-love will allow you to be less self-preoccupied, which will allow you to be more lovingly engaged with life. You will find this a far more relieving and rewarding way to be.

84. Don't run from your "demons." Make them your "friends".

You have a dark side, or shadow side, just like everyone else. Your dark side includes all the things you find unacceptable about yourself. These aren't necessarily bad things. If you feel it is not okay to be assertive and stand out, for example, you may repress these qualities of your character so that they become an unconscious part of your shadow. You then become meek and invisible.

But your soul cannot be denied. Your need to express who you are will seep out around the edges of your ego in the form of unconscious behaviors, anxiety, and depression. By honoring the totality of who you are, you liberate yourself to realize the full expression of who you are. This is an essential part of your healing, for you must be your full, authentic self, regardless of whether you fit in or if it meets with the approval of others—as long as you refrain from intentionally harming others in your quest to be true to yourself.

This brings us to another part of your dark side. This part is the destructive side of you. You, like everyone else, have destructive thoughts, feelings, and urges. You may experience urges to lie to get what you want, or to favorably impress others. You may experience urges to steal. You have likely had urges to take advantage of others, to exploit others for your own personal gain. Perhaps you have experienced the urge to cheat on a test so that you might get a better grade, or to cheat at a game so that you might win. You may have at times experienced urges to hurt others out of anger, or even out of a destructive pleasure in causing harm. Perhaps you have experienced apathy or disregard of the suffering of others. You may have strong competitive urges to win at all costs.

Overcoming these destructive demons starts with radical acceptance of your selfish and destructive thoughts and urges. If you look closely, you will see that you do not directly choose these thoughts and feelings. They are a product of the workings of your brain. Make it a daily practice to not take your brain personally—it is just doing what brains do, and it is not who you are—the Awareness of these thoughts, feelings, and urges. Ironically, accepting your brain function is the first step toward mastering your demons. Change starts with acceptance. You cannot manage what you condemn, repress, or deny. Instead, have compassion for yourself that your brain is generating destructive thoughts and emotions. Your self-compassion will allow for these feelings and urges to pass while you practice lovingly abstaining from acting upon them.

Another demon may be fear. You may fear discomfort, loss, failure, or rejection. Make friends with your fears. They arise out of Mother Nature's protecting you. Fear is good, because it keeps you alive.

If your excessive fears block you from achieving important life goals, your healing will start with not making an enemy out of fear. While fear is very distressing, it is not bad. It is just fear. With this attitude, you can learn to courageously bear your fears while you do what you need to do in life to accomplish your important life goals.

Lastly, there are the demons of addiction and other psychiatric illnesses, such as depression. These are malfunctions of the brain. Befriending your illnesses with compassion for yourself enables you to be loving toward yourself. Love stops you from being in pain about being in pain, thus relieving you of unnecessary suffering. These illnesses will teach you how to learn to live with them and keep them in remission if you honor them. Making an enemy out of your illness puts you in a negative mind state, which is the exact opposite of what you need to heal.

85. Be an ideal parent to yourself.

You didn't grow up with perfectly loving parents who loved you perfectly at all times. None of us had ideal parents. Nor do any of us grow up in ideal societies that lovingly foster our well-being at every turn.

Instead, you were at times hurt, disappointed, and neglected. There may have been times when your parents needed to say "No" to you but they did not. Instead, they may have pushed you to achieve, giving you the subtle message that you were not lovable if you did not live up to their expectations. Society has inundated you with the message that happiness comes from being attractive, successful, or from having pleasurable experiences. All messages such as these can be damaging.

Worse still, you may have suffered from significant emotional or physical neglect, sexual abuse, physical abuse, emotional abuse, or other forms of trauma growing up. If you did, these all significantly damaged your capacity to love.

As a result of the way you were loved by your parents and the way you were treated by society, you likely did not learn how to perfectly love yourself. You have likely developed unloving habits, including addiction.

None of us loves ourselves perfectly at all times. We all do things to harm ourselves, such as not getting enough rest, or working too hard, or working too little, or eating good-tasting foods that are bad for us, or spending too much time on the computer, or not getting enough exercise, and so on.

When you do not take good care of yourself, you harm yourself. To heal, you must start taking very good care of yourself. This is your first act of self-love. This requires that you be your own ideal parent, and treat yourself as if you were your own beloved child.

This will not come naturally, because you will feel an overwhelming urge to do what is familiar to you rather than what is good for you. This is the power of habit. Being your own ideal parent means doing what is best for you regardless of urges to do otherwise. This requires a strong motivation to love yourself in all that you say and do, and the willpower and discipline to carry this through.

Develop loving self-care habits by making small changes in your habits, one at a time, over a period of time. Changing how you live your life doesn't happen overnight.

Start by renouncing all addiction. As your own ideal parent, vow to not harm yourself in any way.

Then, engage in a progressive process of making multiple small changes in how you care for yourself. You might start with getting yourself into a safe place to live and heal. Then care for yourself by surrounding yourself with loving people and asking for their help. Then go on to get adequate rest, nutritious food, and exercise. Brush and floss your teeth daily. Then you might develop a daily spiritual practice. Get the medical and psychiatric care you need to heal. Find something meaningful to do in life that will leave you feeling joyful and fulfilled.

You cannot change the past. But you can make up for the past by being your own ideal parent from this moment on. Realize that no one can do this for you. There is no one who can "fix" you or your life. This is something you must do for yourself, with the help, support, and guidance of others.

86. Seek treatment for medical illnesses so that you can secure your recovery.

If you have any medical illnesses, you will want to get good treatment for them as part of your self-care. The more vital your body is, the more vital your recovery will be. If you are suffering physically, this will add an extra challenge to your recovery. Make your recovery easier by doing what you can to optimize your physical health.

Many people who suffer from narcotic addiction have chronic pain. If this is true for you, then you will need good non-narcotic pain management treatment. This may include non-narcotic analgesics, antidepressants that raise your pain threshold, massage, acupuncture, or physical therapy. Pain psychotherapies exist to also decrease your suffering, as I discussed in a previous lesson. There may be other interventions available to help you. It is best to work with a good pain management practitioner who can coordinate a team effort among multiple providers to help you with your pain.

If you are just getting off opioids now, your physical pain may get worse before it gets better. This is because many people become more sensitive to pain when they take opioids. This is called "opioid-induced hyperalgesia." Narcotics lower your pain threshold. It can take several weeks for your pain threshold to go back up after you stop taking opioids.

If you need to take medications, take them exactly as prescribed. If you have trouble remembering to take your medications, set up a reminder system, such as always taking your medications when you brush your teeth. If you experience medication side effects, contact your prescriber to let them know. Getting the most out of your medical treatment requires taking your medications responsibly.

If you are not happy with your medical treatment, get a second opinion or find a treatment provider who takes a different approach. Medical care is not black and white. Many conditions have more than one treatment approach. You may find you get benefit from working with a holistic provider, a naturopath, a functional medicine specialist, or a traditional medicine provider.

Many medical conditions, such as diabetes, asthma, or high blood pressure, require lifestyle changes as part of their treatment. This might include changes in your nutrition or exercise routines. Work with providers who can help you make positive changes in your daily life habits to optimize your physical health.

87. Seek treatment for psychiatric illnesses to secure your recovery.

You may suffer from depression, anxiety, or some other psychiatric condition. If you do, make sure you get good treatment for all of your psychiatric conditions, not just your addictions.

If possible, try to get treatment for all your psychiatric conditions from one therapist and/or psychiatric prescriber who is competent to treat both your addictions and your other psychiatric conditions. This is easier and more convenient than splitting up your treatment among multiple providers.

Recovery is much more difficult if you are suffering from psychiatric illnesses other than addictions. Other psychiatric illnesses double or triple your suffering and impairment. Recovery is difficult enough work as it is. You will find it even more difficult if you are suffering from impairment due to other psychiatric conditions. This is a good reason why you want to get treatment for everything at once.

Healing and recovery take time. Be patient. It may be difficult at first to cope with cravings to addict and other psychiatric symptoms, such as depression, anxiety, or difficulties thinking clearly. You may have to just persevere with your treatment for a while until you feel better. Have faith and do not give up. You will get better if you continue with your treatment. If you feel hopeless, don't buy into the hopelessness. Feelings can lie. The truth is that your situation is never hopeless, no matter how sick you might be or how badly you have been hurt. It is never hopeless.

When it comes to starting therapy, follow the "three-session rule." If you don't feel helped and hopeful after three sessions, you may want to look for another therapist. Always let your therapist know how you are feeling about the treatment. Don't be shy; remember that they are there to serve you and your needs. You don't need to worry about hurting their feelings. If your therapy isn't going well, talk about it. You may be surprised to find that your therapist responds positively to your concerns and that your therapy takes a turn for the better as a result. If things continue to go poorly after you try to address your concerns, look for another therapist.

Take your therapy seriously. If you are taking medications, take them exactly as prescribed and call your prescriber if you have side effects or other concerns. Don't stop your medications abruptly—that could cause severe withdrawal symptoms and make your original symptoms such as depression or anxiety come back full force. Finding the right antidepressant is a bit of trial and error. Your doctor may ask you to try several medications in order to find the one that is just right for you. The good news is that almost always your doctor and you will figure out a medication regimen that helps.

Many patients hide the complete truth from their therapists out of fear or shame or not wanting to take accountability. Do not hide or distort the truth. Be honest with your therapist. They are there to help you and will not judge you, though they may judge the wisdom or merit of some of your actions. You should feel safe with your therapist to be completely transparent, honest, and authentic. This is incredibly important if they are going to have any chance of helping you.

Your therapist may give you homework, especially if you are receiving treatment to change your thinking and behavior, called "cognitive behavioral therapy" or "CBT." Do your homework diligently. You will not benefit from your therapy if you don't put in the effort. A lot of therapy involves starting to do what is good for you rather than what is familiar to you. This requires effort on your part. If your therapist suggests, for example, that you exercise, meditate, or write in your journal, do these things. Follow through on your therapy agreements. Be diligent. You will be glad you did when you start to feel and function better.

Be receptive and thoughtful if your therapist gives you advice. A good therapist will likely rarely give you advice, unless this advice is obvious, such as to not hang out with people who are addicting. Consider your therapist's advice carefully, but feel free not to follow their advice if it does not feel right for you. It is your life to live. Ultimately you need to go out and live as you best see fit and learn and grow from your mistakes along the way.

88. Learn to manage emotional pain.

People addict to numb pain. You, too, likely used painkillers to numb emotional pain in addition to any physical pain you might have. The central task of healing and recovery is to learn to manage, resolve, and endure emotional pain with loving interventions rather than by numbing pain through addicting. In fact, the secret to a long and successful life is skillful pain management.

Let's talk about how we skillfully manage our emotional pain. The first thing is to not make painful feelings your enemy. You cannot manage your pain if you run from it. Whether you are feeling ashamed, remorseful, hateful, sad, depressed, anxious, angry, lonely, or bored, you must start by having the courage to feel your feelings. They are just feelings, after all. They will not kill you. Not only that, they never last forever. Feelings constantly change.

You may find that you get flooded and overwhelmed if you let yourself feel your pain. If this happens to you, you should work with your therapist on grounding techniques to help you experience your pain without becoming too overwhelmed. This might include breathing and visualization exercises, or other self-soothing mind-body exercises.

Once you can be with and feel your feelings, you can begin to manage them. The first step is to have deep compassion for your suffering. As I emphasized before, this requires that you don't take your brain personally. You are not directly responsible for the thoughts and feelings that arise in your awareness. Painful emotions are a sign that things are not right. Practice deep compassion for yourself if this is the case. Treat yourself the way a loving parent would treat their child.

As you sit with your feelings, you may notice something interesting. You may notice that your feelings give way to deeper, underlying feelings, usually hurt, sadness, or fear.

If you realize you are sad, then maybe you need to cry. If you see that you are afraid, you may need to reassure or console yourself or seek reassurance from others.

Whatever you might be feeling, you need to practice compassionate acceptance of your feelings. You need to allow them to be. Let go of shame, judgment, and resistance.

Once you have embraced your feelings and have shown yourself compassion for your pain, you will likely notice that you feel better already. You just needed to honor how you felt and show yourself some compassion. If you are still sad, hurt, or afraid, you can go about doing things to help yourself feel better. This can include talking out your pain with a loving support person or your therapist. Follow the life rule, "Never hurt alone." A pain shared is a pain halved. Your therapist, friend, or loved one can help you feel better just by showing that they understand how you feel. You will feel better when you are not alone with your pain.

Then you can go about problem solving other ways to feel better. This might include practicing humble acceptance of the way things are, including reverent and radical acceptance of who you are exactly as you are. You may need practice cultivating forgiveness. You may find you feel better if you count your blessings and realize what you are grateful for. You may need to do something to secure your safety if you are legitimately in danger. You might feel better if you do something good or soothing for yourself, such as getting a massage, curling up with a good book, watching a feel-good movie, or taking a walk in nature. Doing something fun or joyful may help you feel better.

Or, you may find you feel better if you do something productive for yourself or for someone you care about. Focusing on loving others is a great way to fill your heart with joy. The options for ways to feel better are many. Whatever your pain, there is a way to either feel better or to make your pain easier to bear.

Recognize emotional pain, accept it, show compassion for your pain, and do things to reduce your pain and cultivate joy. If you follow this pain management strategy, you will gradually replace pain with joy and resolve any cravings to addict.

89. Stress fuels addiction. Learn the skill of managing stress.

Life is difficult and stressful. Stress is inevitable and unavoidable. You will need to skillfully manage your stress to keep addiction at bay. The first step to managing stress is to prevent it if you can. Don't bite off more than you can chew. Live mindfully, with a healthy balance of work, rest, love, and play.

Second, notice when you are stressed. Practice mindfulness. Notice when you feel tense. You cannot address your stress if you do not acknowledge it.

Third, get support. Ask for help. Surround yourself with healthy, loving people. Limit or end relationships with people who are harmful to you.

Fourth, set realistic expectations. Expect life to be an endless series of problems to solve. Expect imperfection and failure. Expect to be wrong much of the time. Acknowledge your limitations. You will be more at peace when you stop expecting yourself or Life to be other than they are. You can do only what you can do. Don't expect more than this.

Fifth, stop worrying about your problems and instead go about solving them. Take action, with the help, guidance, and support of others.

Sixth, prioritize, plan, and pace yourself. You will not achieve all your dreams in one day. Schedule your days, and follow your schedule. Deal with first things first. Don't go too slow, but don't go too fast. Take breaks and rest along the way.

Seventh, engage in surrendered action. This means doing your best, hoping for a good outcome, but accepting what is beyond your control. You can't control what other people think, say, or do, for example, even though you might have tremendous influence over others. Do your best and accept the rest.

Eighth, relax, release, and reset. Sometimes the most effective way to solve a big problem is to take a break from it and do something else. Engage in a daily practice of silence and stillness. Practice deep, mindful breathing and muscle relaxation techniques. Take time-outs. Get outside in nature.

Ninth, take very good care of yourself. As mentioned earlier, eat healthfully, get plenty of sleep, keep a regular routine, exercise, have fun, and love others. All of these actions will help to keep you vital so that you can weather stress.

Tenth, keep a healthy perspective. Stay realistic, positive, and hopeful. Ask yourself what this problem will mean 1,000 years from now. Keep in mind that the Universe is rigged in your favor if you just maintain your hope and act skillfully. Remember that attitude is everything, including an attitude of gratitude. Stay grateful during tough times for your many blessings. Also remind yourself that just as good times never last, so do hard times always pass. Sometimes what is needed is just putting one foot in front of the other and forging ahead.

These ten "stress busters" will help keep you happy, healthy, and in recovery during the many hard times ahead. Make them part of your daily habit of living.

90. Understand your own values. Make sure they are healthy for you.

A great deal of unnecessary suffering and unskillful behavior result from unhealthy values. Having the right values to guide your behavior will help you to heal and realize a joyful life. Your values represent what is important to you. You can tell your values from your behavior. What you do and how you live directly reflect what is important to you. Examples of values include:

- Spirituality
- Family
- Honesty
- Success
- Faithfulness
- Accountability
- Dependability
- Dignity
- Responsibility
- Intelligence
- Self-esteem
- Intimacy
- Career
- Being accepted
- Wealth
- Pleasure
- Fun
- Popularity
- Happiness
- Generosity
- Cooperation
- Personal peace
- God's will
- Growth
- Humility
- Forgiveness
- Candor
- Commitment
- Honor
- Achievement
- Leadership
- Love
- Independence
- Fitting in
- Attractiveness
- Adventure
- Being respected
- Freedom
- Power
- Compassion
- Creativity

There are literally hundreds of values. Some of them come from ego concerns for safety, comfort, survival, power, and status. Some of them come from love-based Higher Self concerns such as forgiveness, honesty, intimacy, generosity, and contentment.

Think about the value, "He who dies with the most toys wins." Someone who believes this sees life as a competition, where there are winners and losers. This person also believes that material wealth is what makes a person a "winner." Materialism is an example of an unhealthy value. Look around you. See that despite our material wealth and comfort, the suicide rate continues to rise and our country is in the grips of an addiction epidemic.

Another unhealthy value that you may hold is that the meaning of life is to have as many pleasurable experiences as possible and as little pain as possible. This is understandable, as we all want to feel good and not feel bad. Yet gratification and relief of pain are the values that led you into addiction.

Another unhealthy value is the feeling that it is important that you are popular. If your goal in life is for other people to like you, you will twist yourself into a pretzel of inauthenticity in order to glean the approval of others. Since mental health entails being true to yourself while respecting the rights of others, needing too much for others to like you will tie the hands of your soul and make you spiritually ill. Your ego watches out for your safety, security, and status. When you're at risk of being rejected, you will need to look carefully at the person or group that is rejecting you. Do you share their values? Have you behaved in some unskillful or destructive way? If not, then needing too much to be liked may be a compromise of your integrity.

Another, more sneaky, unhealthy value is the need to be successful to feel okay about yourself. This value says that your value as a person is based upon your performance, and not on the fact that you are a human being. Although achieving things is great, needing to achieve to feel good about yourself is not great. First of all, it makes an enemy out of failure, when in fact failure is your friend. If you are no good if you fail, then how are you going to fail so that you can grow?

Take a good, long look at your values. To do this, carefully examine your behavior. Your behavior does not lie. Don't let yourself fool yourself. See the real truth of things—what your values truly are. Then ask yourself if these values serve your happiness, joy, and serenity. If not, then it is time to do some contemplation on what values would truly serve you.

What values would serve you? How about honesty? How about being a good friend, spouse, family member? How about being true to your soul? What about putting in a good day's work for a good day's pay? What about making your peace with being an imperfect person just like everyone else?

Above all, there are two things we all should value the most. One is this precious gift of life. We should value the opportunity to savor the gift of existence. Out of your valuing your life, you will do everything you can to enhance your well-being and vitality. This is what it means to love yourself. Second, we should value the opportunity to love others and be of service in some way according to our gifts and what the world asks of us. In the end, what matters most in life is that we love ourselves, love others, and love Life itself. Love is the highest of values.

91. Self-compassion is part of good self-care.

If you're like most people who suffer from addiction, you are pretty hard on yourself. You may even hate yourself. Trauma and neglect growing up have a way of doing this to us.

Unfortunately, self-hatred is pretty common in our narcissistic culture. It starts with the fact that we all automatically compare ourselves to others. We notice who is the brightest, who is the most athletic, who is the prettiest or most handsome, who has a lot of money, who is the most popular, who went to the best schools, and so on. This is just what humans do. What is unhealthy is that we buy into these beliefs and either feel badly about ourselves when we come up short or feel superior to others when we come out on top. Then we feel either self-hatred or arrogance, neither of which is good for us.

The problem is that hating yourself is not good for you, even if you feel you deserve it. It won't make you a better person. Instead, it will just fuel your addiction.

The way to heal is to show yourself compassion when you are suffering. If you want to heal and realize your full potential, you need to start by loving yourself, even with your addiction. You need to be very kind to yourself when you are in pain, including when you find yourself hating yourself.

Showing yourself compassion has many benefits. It helps you to feel better. It helps you to heal. Ironically, it helps you to change, because change starts with compassionate self-acceptance. This is not to say that you don't hold yourself accountable for your behavior. You do. But you also show yourself compassion for your suffering. Self-compassion improves your accountability, because you can own your behavior without beating yourself up.

Self-compassion is good for others as well. When you are compassionate to yourself, your compassion extends outward to others, improving your relationships with them.

Cultivate self-compassion through practice. First, practice unconditional kindness toward yourself at all times, no matter how badly you screw up. Judge your actions to be unskillful, but never judge your personhood. Say to yourself, "I'm sorry you're having a hard time" and renounce ever treating yourself harshly. That is simply not a loving thing to do to anyone, including yourself.

Second, see that you are ultimately no different from anyone else, except perhaps in degrees. You are not alone. See that everyone suffers, and that everyone is imperfect. We are all beautiful bozos on the bus, each one of us just doing the best we can at this moment. You didn't choose the cards you were dealt, and you're just trying to figure out how to play them as best you can, just like everyone else. Seeing that everyone is struggling, just as you are, will help you to give yourself a break.

Third, practice being aware of your pain and your self-hatred. Watch for it like a guard at the gate to a fort. Notice as soon as you can when you are suffering so that you can practice compassion for yourself. Notice and immediately let go of harsh self-criticism and self-judgment. Say something kind to yourself when you notice you are starting to beat yourself up. Self-hatred is a very bad mental habit that will require intentional effort on your part to recognize and correct, over and over again for a lifetime.

All people are worthy of being loved. This means you are worthy of being loved by yourself. It doesn't matter how awful you think you are—those are just negative, toxic thoughts. Sure, you're imperfect and have problems. Welcome to the human race. Make a commitment, starting right now, to do two things. The first is to act with love in all you say and do, to everyone and to yourself. The more loving you are, the more lovable you will feel. The second is to be very kind to yourself when you are in pain or when any sort of negative self-evaluations arise.

Neutralize these toxic thoughts and feelings with unconditional kindness. These practices will create the conditions for healing and recovery to occur.

92. Learn to forgive.

Forgiveness of both yourself and others is good for you. Forgiveness will help you to heal by releasing the pain of self-condemnation, hatred, and resentment.

You've probably been hurt, maybe even a lot, by many people. You've probably also hurt a lot of people as well. If so, your mind may be filled with bitterness and resentment toward others along with self-condemnation. These negative emotional states will only fuel readdicting. You will need to dissolve bitterness and resentment to fully heal.

You can't really decide to forgive. Forgiveness is something that happens when you create the right conditions for forgiveness to occur. Here's what you should practice to allow for forgiveness to arise:

- *Practice humility.* See that you are flawed, just like everyone else. Let go of any grandiose need to be perfect. This will help you to not be so hard on yourself. Instead, nurture an authentic wish to be decent.

- *Practice understanding.* See that our selfish, hurtful, and addictive behaviors stem from pain and ignorance. See that the neglect and abuse we suffered can condition us to be neglectful and abusive. See that all of us, including you, have a dark side not of our choosing. Everyone is driven by fear and desire that can trigger us to disregard the needs of others. See how easy it can be for you and others to be selfish and hurtful.

- *Imagine yourself or the person you resent as being a child.* How would you treat a child? See that we all were once innocent. Reflect on the fact that no one chooses their genes, their character, their parents, or their environment growing up. See that if you were the person who hurt you, you may well have acted exactly as they did.

- *Reflect on the harm you have done to others.* Recognize that everyone has done harm to others.
  - ° As you consider your harmful behavior, contemplate the role of your disease or ignorance in your actions. Your understanding will promote compassion for yourself.
  - ° As you consider others' harmful behavior, contemplate the role of their disease, ignorance, or situation in their actions. Your understanding will promote compassion for others.
- *Pray (in a way that is meaningful for you) for the person who has harmed you.* Pray for yourself. This invites forgiveness.
- *Give something to the person you resent.* Perhaps a gift of something that they need. Pick up something for them from the store. Do something for them, like bringing in the trash cans for your neighbor. Give them a call to check in on how they are doing. It is difficult to resent someone when you are giving to them.
- *See that your resentment arises from unrealistic expectations of yourself and others.* Accept people as they are and Reality as it is—a perfectly imperfect Universe that only seems imperfect from our limited point of view. Accept others while still holding them accountable for their actions.
- *See your role, if any, in the harm done to you.* This practice takes courage and honesty. How might you have put yourself in harm's way?
- *Remember the sacredness of all things.* All people are sacred and deserving of your respect and reverence due to the mere fact they exist, even with their destructive sides. This may be difficult for you to accept. It is easier if you're able to see your own destructiveness and if you recognize that all things and all people are perfectly imperfect and can only be as they are.

- *Let go of injured pride.* It was never about you in the first place. Treat others with respect and care because you are a respectful and caring person.

- *See life as an opportunity for growth, liberation, and a deepening of your humility rather than focusing on whether you are being rewarded, harmed, or punished.* Don't focus on what you're getting or not getting from others. Instead, focus on how you can become a more loving person and have more peace of mind.

- *Contemplate the fact that resentment and self-condemnation hurt you.* Ask yourself if your resentments and self-condemnation bring you joy or pain.

Forgiveness does not mean letting other people or yourself off the hook. We are all still accountable for our behavior and for the consequences of our behavior. It also does not mean that you necessarily have a relationship with someone who has harmed you. You need to protect yourself from harm even while you practice forgiveness.

Forgiveness of yourself and others will lighten your heart and promote your recovery. Do what you can to assert yourself and protect yourself from future harm. Through your practice of forgiveness, may you move into your recovery with a loving heart and a protective emotional shield.

93. Develop a hobby.

Is there some hobby that you've always thought about, but never acted on? This is a good time to explore. Joyful and meaningful engagement in life takes away cravings to addict. This is because you are so caught up in enjoying what you are doing that your brain feels less of a need for something more.

If you can create one or two projects that you feel passionate about, these projects will do two things. First, they will take up your time. The more you are actually involved with a project, the less idle time you will have to think about addicting.

Second, your projects will provide you with many rewards. You'll have the reward of doing something meaningful. Or, it may be rewarding because it is fun. Maybe you'll have the reward of doing something challenging. You may experience the reward of doing something creative. Then there is the reward of achieving something difficult. You may experience the reward of solving a difficult problem or making a meaningful contribution to your community. Whatever the rewards, in the end, your passions and projects will be fulfilling as they serve as a way to enjoy life.

Remember that it is not gratification that will secure your recovery. It is fulfillment. Doing things that are meaningful and fulfilling are the most satisfying.

This is not to say there is anything wrong with having fun. Fun is good, too. If you can find things to do that are fun, challenging, and meaningful, you've got it made!

So what should you do? There are literally millions of options. You could do volunteer work, take up a sport, join a group, play an instrument, become a craft maker, or do any of thousands of other things. The ideal is to do something you enjoy. It helps if you also have a talent for it. If it serves a need, even better, because you'll have the fulfillment of contributing.

Let's imagine that you enjoy reading. You could join a book club. You might also volunteer to read to senior citizens in a local nursing home, or help young people learn to read at your nearby school. In this example, you're doing something you enjoy, getting social contact, and maybe helping other people all at the same time.

Your passions and projects should be active, not passive. They should require action and effort. You are better off avoiding passive activities such as watching TV. While TV may numb and distract you, if will not fulfill you.

While solitary passions such as painting, coin collecting, or model building can be satisfying, passions and projects that bring you together into community with others add an extra dimension of meaning.

We humans are designed to be active. We are also designed to invest ourselves in things outside of ourselves. When you do, you feel fulfilled. The more fulfilled you feel, the less you will feel the need for the "something more" that you feel in the emptiness of addiction.

If you have things you'd like to start doing, great! Schedule them into your week and get going. If you're not sure what you'd like to do, then do some brainstorming. Talk with others about what you might do. You can even look up things to do on the Internet.

94. Practice stillness through prayer, meditation, or contemplation.

Everything in your life and in your recovery begins and ends with your spirituality. I've talked about spirituality and spiritual practices in previous lessons. In this lesson, I want to focus on the importance of stillness for your healing. When you are still, you are awake. The thought chatter of the monkey mind dies down, and you experience Reality directly, fully, and freshly.

Stillness promotes the experience of unity. Your spiritual experiences of oneness, unity, love, and the sacredness of your life and of all of existence color everything you think, feel, and do. When you are spiritually healthy, you feel a deep sense of connectedness to a loving and sacred Reality. Your sense of your identity expands to include those around you. You feel your goodness and perfection as part of one good and perfect Universe. You experience a sense of peace, even in the midst of the many difficulties and painful experiences of life.

Stillness promotes a sense of the Sacred. Love arises from stillness. This will protect you from addicting. You know that this moment is sacred just as it is, and that you are sacred just as you are. Harming yourself by addicting is not only not necessary, it is just not an option, as you will do nothing to harm yourself or others. Stillness inspires a profound reverence and respect for yourself, for others, and for all of Life. Reverence and respect neutralize cravings.

Stillness promotes peace. When you get very still, there is a feeling that all is well beneath the surface of your troubled emotions. Stillness is like a container of love and peace that can hold all your negative feelings, including feelings of anger, shame, fear, loneliness, or self-hatred.

Attaining and maintaining this state of awakened consciousness requires the regular, daily practice of stillness. Spiritual practices concentrate and still the mind so that you can experience Awareness before thought. Spiritual practices take you out of your immersion in your thinking mind so that you can experience Reality directly. These practices help you to wake up and see the obvious before you that was clouded by your ego—that sense of "I" existing as a separate self, apart from everything else.

Stillness practices help you to see, for example, that you are the Universe aware of Itself, a concept I discussed earlier: Your life and all of life are both a blessing and a miracle. Awakened by your practice, you experience the inspiration to dedicate your life to both nurturing life and savoring this brief, precious, momentary gift of existence.

You can enter stillness and awaken through many practices, including meditation, yoga, qigong (a Chinese practice of breathing, movement, and meditation), tai chi, centering prayer, and contemplation. I've touched on some of these practices in a previous lesson.

Stillness is like a refuge you can return to over and over again as you experience the storms of daily life. It is always there for you. All you have to do is get still and present. Stop as often as necessary, especially when you are feeling emotionally aroused. Take a deep breath, concentrate on this moment, asking yourself, "What is this?" Then sink into the quiet depths of your still Awareness beneath the surface ripples of experience (your thoughts and feelings). When you are still, you know who you truly are.

Stillness will not only protect your recovery, it will also enhance the quality of each day. You will feel more peaceful, calmer, more grounded, clearer, and more centered. You will move through your days with more wisdom, compassion, and skill. You will also notice life to be a bit more vibrant. You will experience more positive emotions, such as joy, gratitude, love, and wonder.

Also, you will notice your tolerance of pain and distress will go up. The rewards of a practice of stillness are many. You want to make the best of this one precious life you have been given. Make the best of it by starting your day in stillness, carrying stillness into the motion of your day, and ending your day in stillness.

95. Visualize what you want in life.

Positive change starts with a positive vision of the life you want. When you visualize yourself actually living the life you want, you activate some of the same networks of brain cells that would activate if your dreams were reality. By visualizing, you prime your brain to act to make your dreams come true. Some say visualization activates our creative unconscious. Visualization is part of the process of creation.

What you visualize, you eventually express through action. True to the Law of Attraction, the Universe resonates with the positive energy you put out. It gives back to you that positive energy from others. This is how visualization causes you to attract to you what you want.

What you can conceive and believe, you can achieve. This is why professional athletes use visualization to improve their performance. Similarly, visualizing your dream life improves your performance in making your dream life a reality. Visualization helps you to design your life with clarity and purpose. Visualization also increases motivation to act to achieve your dreams. It inspires you to put in the necessary effort and initiative to make it happen.

Below are some guides to visualization. Do your visualization exercise first thing in the morning. Get still, calm, and present, so that you can practice with mindfulness. You want a still, present mind for these exercises to be effective.

- Before you start, write down your life meaning and purpose, as well as your key life goals. Think about what you want more of in your life. Is it freedom, love, friends, health, happiness, joy, adventure, losing weight, or inner peace? You must know what you want before you can visualize it to achieve it.

- After you have written your life meaning and purpose and key life goals, write a description of the circumstances of your life and the qualities of being that you want to realize. Play with them. Modify them until you have a clear, written statement of your total life vision.

- Now, use your journal to write the story of how your ideal life will come to be. How are you making that ideal a reality? How are you living today to create your ideal life tomorrow?

○ What are your daily rituals and practices?

○ How are you taking care of yourself?

○ What are you doing every day to achieve your life vision?

○ How are you improving your relationships?

○ In addition to visualizing your dream life, you also want to visualize how you are going to spend each day to realize your key life goals.

• After you have written out the story of your dream life, you might want to create a vision board, with pictures that represent you achieving your dreams. Look at your board daily.

• To start the visualization practice, get somewhere safe and quiet, without distractions and interruptions.

• Start by settling yourself and grounding yourself in your body. Take a few deep breaths and focus on your breath. Get still. Center yourself. Let your thinking mind quiet. Visualizations are most effective after meditation or prayer. In visualization, you replace attending to the breath with attending to an inner mental image.

• Take about five to ten minutes for this exercise. Close your eyes. Use all your senses to create a whole life vision in your mind. What do you see, hear, taste, smell, feel, and think? Where are you? What are you doing? Play out your day. Who are you with? Visualize your life as a movie of which you are a key actor. This is called having an "embodied image." Experience everything in as much vivid detail as possible.

• Visualize your life meaning and purpose. What is it like to be living out that purpose?

• Visualize yourself realizing your key life goals. Visualize that you already have what you desire. Practice repeatedly over time to make this as real as possible.

- In your mind, experience what it feels like right now to be your ideal you living your ideal life. Visualize in the Present, not the future. Visualize the results of your efforts. Feel the emotions you will experience when you realize your dreams. They may include satisfaction, contentment, love, joy, appreciation, or gratitude. Hold on to these feelings as you go about your day. Remember that what you put out, you get back. That's how Reality operates. If you want love in your life, for example, be the love you want to attract. Visualize it, and live it throughout the day through your affirmations and intentions.

- Be true to yourself. Visualize being your authentic self, living out your gifts based on your temperament. For example, if you are an introvert who likes time alone, don't force yourself to visualize hopping from one social engagement to another. Visualize the life that will truly fulfill you, not a life you think you should have.

- Visualize the positive. Visualize what you want, not what you don't want. See yourself doing positive things rather than not doing negative things.

- Imagine every step of a healthy activity or interaction. This could include eating, working out, talking with others, doing what you love. Visualize as much detail as possible what you are doing from the start of your day to the end.

- Repeat. Practice. Do this exercise one to three times a day, for five to ten minutes, every day. Remember that the brain needs repetition to change.

- Some people write out thirty to forty key life goals they want to accomplish on index cards. Then they visualize completing each one for several seconds each morning and night. This is another way to practice this visualization exercise.

- Now go out and put your vision into practice. Translate your vision, affirmations, and intentions into a daily life practice of acting to make your vision a reality.

End your visualization exercise with the repetition of affirmations and intentions. Expect to have difficulties with this exercise at first. Give it time and repetition. You will get into a good groove after about thirty days. Have faith and don't give up. New habits take effort, discipline, and faith to develop. If it is hard at first, reassure yourself that it will get easier in about two weeks. Your visualization capabilities will improve with practice. Change does not happen overnight. But change will occur with practice. You won't experience the benefits without daily practice. Change requires repetition. Practice with patience and persistence. Give yourself about ninety days to begin to see the results of your practice. Notice how your practice changes your actions during the day. Then notice how your actions change your life. Remember, be positive, patient, and persistent. If you make the effort, the results will be yours in time.

96. Practice daily affirmations and decide what your intentions are.

After you have written out your life vision and key life goals, you need to go about making your dream life a reality. This requires daily, positive, purposeful action.

Negative, self-limiting beliefs will hinder your realization of your ideal life vision. Counter negative, self-limiting beliefs with the daily practice of positive affirmations. State your intentions to act to make your affirmations a reality. Affirmations coupled with intentions, or commitments, lead to action, which leads to results. By repeating positive affirmations, you re-program your subconscious mind to counter negative, self-limiting beliefs.

Affirmations can transform your life. Words have power. What you voice, you attract. What you say is what you get. You need to express the reality you want to have. When you do, your unconscious mind inspires and motivates you to act to make your affirmations a reality.

Include the following elements in each of your affirmations:

- State positive affirmations in the present tense. The brain works in the Present. "I have," or "I am." Not "I will be."

- Effective affirmations are relevant to your current situation and relate to the key life goals you wish to achieve.

- Positive affirmations include only positive words. The brain can't easily process negatives, such as "I am not fat." Instead, say, "I am becoming fit and trim."

- Positive affirmations are spoken as statements of truth.

- Affirmations are realistic. Your affirmation voices what you can be and do today. Don't make affirmations that are not in accordance with what you can put into practice today. For example, avoid affirmations such as "I am a millionaire" when that is not the case. Instead, you might say, "I am working to double my income over the next year."

- Make your affirmations active, not passive. For example, rather than saying "money flows to me," say, "I work hard and exercise my creativity to find ways to increase my income."

It's okay if your affirmations are not the truth of who you were yesterday. Affirmations are effective when, through your intentions, you can realize them today.

Couple each affirmation with an intention. Your intentions are action statements that result from your affirmations. Through your intentions, you put your affirmations into action to realize your life vision. You actualize your Higher Self through your intentions. Affirmations followed by intentions influence your actions, which then influence your outcomes. Positive intentions produce positive actions, which produce positive results.

When you say your affirmations and intentions, say them like you mean them. Say them with conviction, authority, and belief. What you believe creates your reality. Say them out loud, with all your heart. Feel them when you say them. Capture the feeling of what you are trying to manifest. Do them in front of the mirror, while looking yourself directly in the eyes. Get still, calm, and mindfully present before you say them.

The more you say your affirmations and intentions, the more you will believe them. The more you believe them, the more you will act on them through your daily intentions. Through your actions, your reality will begin to change. Everything you do starts with an intention. An intention triggers each decision and every action you take. Your actions then shape your destiny. Good intentions lead to good results, while bad intentions lead to bad results. This is karma. Good intentions create the conditions for wholesome consequences.

Set intentions to act and be a certain way based upon what matters most to you, in alignment with your values. Live grounded in your good intentions to bolster your integrity and the quality of your life.

Base your intentions on your affirmations. Make your intentions an expectation of how you will act today. Be realistic, however. You may want to start small and build from there. Go up in achievable, incremental steps.

Make intentions positive actions—things you will do. So, rather than saying, "Today, I will not gossip," say, "Today, I will speak only good of others."

You can make affirmations and set intentions in virtually any area of your life, including love, relationships, physical health, money, and values. See the sample list of affirmations and intentions in the Appendix of this book. Here is an example of an affirmation and intention on recovery:

"I am living a joyful life free of addiction. Today I will go to a recovery meeting, talk with my recovery mentor, and call someone whenever cravings arise."

Change requires support. You will benefit from an accountability partner for keeping to your intentions. You will be more likely to keep your commitments if you share them with someone else. Share your intentions for the day with someone. You may even hire a coach or a trainer to keep you accountable.

Actions shape your life. If you start the day with visualizing the life you want as if it were real today, followed by reciting positive affirmations and then reinforcing your affirmations with intentions, you will eventually start acting on those intentions. Then, your positive actions will lead to positive results. As you change on the inside, your life will change on the outside.

97. Express gratitude.

Happiness researchers have found that two things that increase happiness are mindfulness and gratitude. Focusing on what you are grateful for is powerful—it brings you into the here and now. Gratitude helps you in your recovery by countering negative emotional states that bring on addicting.

Gratitude does not come naturally. Our minds have a tendency to focus on the few things that are wrong rather than on the many things that are right. We are biased toward the negative. If we were on an island paradise, we would quickly start complaining about the heat or the mosquitoes.

Not only that, we quickly get used to what is good in our lives and take it for granted. If you stop and think about it, the fact that you are alive and are reading these words is nothing short of a miracle. Yet how often do you wake up in the morning amazed that you have the gift of yet another day of conscious, self-aware existence? If you didn't wake up this morning feeling this way, you've gotten used to the miraculous.

When you are spiritually healthy, you have this amazing moment of conscious awareness that is abundantly more than enough to be pleased with life. But this is not how the ego works. The ego wants more, and more, and more. We all suffer from "Never Enough" syndrome that poisons our gratitude.

You probably have a lot of pain and difficulties in your life that can make gratitude difficult. You may have suffered from a lot of trauma and maybe neglect growing up. If you're like most people with addiction, you probably have a long list of problems you have to deal with. You may also be living in very difficult or even toxic circumstances. You may be filled with hatred and resentment toward the many people who have harmed or neglected you. If these things are true for you, know that an intentional practice of gratitude is crucial to help you endure your adversity. It is especially important that you cultivate an attitude of gratitude to help you overcome all that lies before you and all the pain and trauma that you have already suffered.

Counter your negativity and protect your recovery with a daily, intentional practice of gratitude. You will have to do this with purpose, because gratitude rarely arises spontaneously on its own. It's just not in our nature to be grateful.

Start with gratitude for the basic conditions that allow for life on this planet. Give thanks for the air you breathe, for clean water, and for the life-giving energy of the sun. Be grateful for the earth and the rain, which give forth the life that sustains you. Be grateful for the dynamic web of life that provides you with food to eat.

Then do a gratitude review of your body. If you can see, be grateful you can see. If you can hear, be grateful you can hear. If you can move your body, be grateful for that. Reflect on the millions of processes occurring in your body right now, beyond your control, so that you can live. Couple your gratitude with wonder and amazement at the incredible intelligence of nature that brings you to life.

Now reflect upon the literally millions and millions of people over the many thousands of years who all contributed to your experience of this moment, to the civilization that you enjoy, to the house you are in, to the education you received, to the clothes you wear, and to the food you eat. No matter how horrific your past might have been, you would not be here now if it were not for the generosity, sustenance, and love of many people, most of whom you will never know.

Finally, reflect on the reality of healing and grace. Other people with severe addiction have survived, healed, and gone on to thrive. Feel grateful that you, too, have this opportunity. Think about the recovery supports and treatment resources available to you to help you recover from your illness and trauma. Have gratitude that you have this chance to live a better life than you have lived up until now.

I'm sure that if you thought about it you could come up with a list of hundreds of reasons to be grateful. Make a gratitude list, and slowly add to it every time you think of something you appreciate that either happened in the past or that you have now.

Gratitude is a balm for the wounds of bitterness and despair. Apply it generously on a daily basis to your life. When you do, you will notice a deepening of your joy.

98. Journaling can deepen insight.

The benefits of keeping a daily journal are many. To begin, journaling brings to the surface what lies just below your awareness. Journaling brings focus and clarity to your life. It allows you to go deeper into the truth of your existence. In this way, journaling promotes insight and wisdom.

Journaling gives you a safe, private forum in which to work out solutions to your daily dilemmas. You can invoke the "Wise Person" within you, writing about how he or she would solve a particular problem. You will often find yourself amazed at the wisdom you discover within yourself through journaling.

In the busyness of life, you probably have many moments when fleeting insights come and go. Journaling gives you the opportunity to stop, take a time-out from the rush of life, and delve into contemplation and reflection in order to capture and flesh out these insights. Journaling forces a pause for reflection.

Journaling is a great way to work on cravings, especially if you don't have a recovery support available with whom you can talk out your cravings. Instead, you can write them out. Write about the good things that will likely occur if you don't addict and the bad things that will likely occur if you do addict. Then, see if you can write about what might have triggered your cravings. It may be people, places, or things that reminded you of using, or it might have been a painful emotion. If you are hurting, write about why you are hurting. Then, write about the things you are going to do to help yourself feel better. Just writing about and acknowledging your pain with compassion for yourself can be incredibly therapeutic if it is coupled with ways to help yourself feel better.

If someone has hurt you, you might want to write them a letter in your journal telling them how they harmed you. Just writing out your pain helps you to bear and release your pain. You don't need to mail the letter, just write out your thoughts and feelings. Journaling is a great way to learn from your experience. If you slip, for example, use your journal to explore what happened. Write about the sequence of events, the circumstances, the thoughts and feelings that triggered the slip. Write about what you did and what you should have done differently, and why you didn't do what you should have. In this way, the clarity of your writing will propel your learning and growth.

If you have a dilemma, journal about it. Write it out. Write about all the possible options for dealing with your problem, and all the pros and cons of each option. Sometimes writing about your problems in this way will give you clarity on how to resolve them.

Go over your journal entries with your recovery mentor or other loving and wise recovery supports. Their feedback and insights will enhance the benefits of journaling.

If you're not in the habit of journaling, you will need to work on making it a habit. The way to do this is to reflect on all the benefits of journaling so that you want to do it. Then, to make it easy for yourself, start by journaling for one to five minutes a day just to get the habit going. Then, set up a trigger for journaling. This could be brushing your teeth at night before bed or getting a cup of coffee in the morning. Every time you brush your teeth, for example, your next act would be to journal for a few minutes, even if just to write a sentence or two about how your day went. Try this for a few months and see how you like it. If it benefits you, the benefits should motivate you to keep it up.

99. Reading will benefit your recovery.

You likely already know the benefits of reading because you are reading this book. Keep it up! Reading will greatly benefit your recovery. Literally thousands of gifted people have written thousands of great books on recovery, healing, and optimal living. The amount of insight and wisdom available to you is vast. Never before have so many useful books been so readily available. You could literally read every day, all day, for the rest of your life, and not begin to get through all the available literature. One of the things that is great about this is the diversity of insights, opinions, and perspectives out there on any given topic. When it comes to food for thought, there is a feast awaiting you!

You can read some books quickly, while you will benefit from reading others slowly and thoughtfully. This can be especially true for reading spiritual literature. For these, it is often helpful to read a passage and then pause to contemplate the passage, going deep into the meaning of the text and how it relates to your life.

Make it a habit to read with a highlighter or pen in hand. Mark important passages and write notes to yourself in the margins. Then, when you are done, go back and read through what you have marked and written. This will help cement what you have read in your memory.

Another good practice is to talk about what you are reading with a friend, family member, or recovery support. This also helps to solidify your learning. It might also inspire conversation or debate with others that will further deepen your understanding.

You will come across some books that are timeless classics. Make it a habit to reread these books from time to time, perhaps every few years or so. One example for me is *The Road Less Traveled* by M. Scott Peck. This is a great book that discusses love and spirituality in the process of healing and transformation.

You may want to join or start a book club. Do you have any other friends in recovery who like to read? Do you know of any book clubs in your area? Book clubs are a great way to enjoy a book with others, giving you a social outlet as well as a way to dive deep into a book.

Twelve-step groups often have "Big Book" meetings. Members read and discuss sections out of texts such as *Narcotics Anonymous* in these meetings. In a way, these groups are a little like Bible studies. They help members to get the most out of these rich texts.

Reading will broaden your horizons, deepen your insight, inspire you, and give you invaluable guidance on this life's journey. You should make daily reading part of your regular recovery routine.

As with journaling, develop a habit of reading by starting small. You might want to keep a book by your journal, and commit to reading one page a day or even just one paragraph a day. Another great technique to consider is to first read a small passage and then write about it in your journal, linking what you read, if possible, to the realities of your life. In this way, reading and journaling come together as a great combination for enhancing your recovery and your life.

100. Exercise is good for the mind and body.

We all know exercise is good for us. Yet few of us actually get regular exercise. But did you know that exercise is good for you both physically *and* mentally? It is true. Exercise relieves stress and promotes a positive outlook on life. Not only does exercise increase strength, stamina, and the length of your life, it also increases the quality of your emotional life as well. This includes increasing your resistance to triggers and cravings to readdict. You can promote your recovery through regular exercise.

I like to exercise mindfully, focusing all my attention on running, or lifting weights. I combine meditation and exercise. Often, I will count my breaths as I am running, starting over when a thought arises. At the end of a workout session, this leaves me with a good feeling. I feel calm, refreshed, relaxed, and centered. It is a great way to start the day.

Here are a few tips and tricks to help you get into a regular exercise routine:

- *Schedule your exercise.* Build it into your day. It likely won't happen if you don't schedule it. Then, make it one of your high priorities, right up there with your recovery meetings and other recovery rituals.

- *Do things you like.* That could include hiking, or playing tennis, or going surfing. You are more likely to exercise if it is fun.

- *Consider getting an exercise partner.* This person will help keep you accountable and on track. They also make exercising more fun.

- *Another option is to get a trainer.* Trainers not only help keep you exercising regularly, they also guide you along the way. Trainers are especially useful if you have never exercised before.

- *Mix it up.* Run one day, bike another, swim another. Mix cardio with weight training. You may want to alternate what you do on different days. You will get the most out of your exercise if you do a variety of things.

- *Start small and don't overdo it.* If you can exercise for just twenty minutes a day, that is a great start. If you are out of shape, start low and go slow. You don't want to injure yourself.

- *Be consistent.* Barring life emergencies, try to keep to your schedule. Try as much as possible to not let life get in the way. To benefit the most from exercise, you should exercise consistently.

- *If you don't feel like exercising, focus on how good you will feel when you are done.* Invariably, you will feel refreshed when you are done, even if you go into exercising feeling tired and stressed out.

- *Set up a reward system for yourself.* For example, you can make a deal with a friend to go out for dinner or to a movie once a week for every week that you exercise five times a week.

Make exercise a regular life habit. It will not only benefit your recovery, it will likely add years to your life and life to your years.

101. Be authentic and true to yourself.

Every day, there are people everywhere telling you what and how to be. This is called "socialization." Growing up, people likely praised and punished you a lot in order to get you to "be good" and to "behave." Some of this was good, as you had to learn how to be safe and how to respect the rights of others. Some of it may have been harmful if it made you feel bad about yourself.

Then, in your preteen and teen years, you experienced enormous pressures from your peers to "be cool" and to "fit it." You may have even felt pressure not to "be different" or to be "like everyone else." Being sensitive to rejection, you either found a group of friends where you could fit in or, if you felt like an outcast, you soothed the pain of rejection somehow, perhaps by using drugs.

With the drive to be included comes the drive to have status. We are bombarded by society's messages about who is the prettiest, the most handsome, the smartest, the strongest, the most athletic, the richest, the coolest, and so on. In our narcissistic society, everybody wants to be special. If you feel you're average or below average, like most of us, you can end up feeling pretty miserable about yourself.

Society is telling you every day, in every way, not only how to think, feel, and act, but also what you're worth. I'm sure you can relate to these pressures. We all feel them. It can put us in a bind, because if we are truly authentic and true to the callings of our souls, we risk both criticism and rejection if we don't fit in.

One of the hardest things you'll have to do in life is to figure out how to be both authentically who you are while being interdependent with others. You can think of this as the paradox of autonomy and interdependence. It is a difficult riddle to solve. How do you live true to your own nature while respecting and even nurturing family, friends, and all the other people in your life? The following guidelines work for me:

- *Listen to your soul.* Honor your intuitions and gut feelings. Pay attention to your dreams. Consider carefully what others say and do and what they ask of you. Respond with care for what is right and best for you and others. Live a thoughtful, reflective life in which you consider carefully what is true, right, and good for you and others. Live from your Higher Self while honoring your survival needs.

- *Beware of self-delusion.* It is so easy to fool ourselves. Be wary of your motivations. Live with humility. Ask yourself why you are doing what you are doing. Be mindful of your ego. You will know it is at work when you feel fear, anger, insufficiency, or some other desire for self-enhancement. If you feel these forces at work, stop and be very honest with yourself about them. Then honor your feelings while asking yourself, "What would love do?"

- *Live and let live.* Just as I don't want anyone telling me what I should do or how I should be, so I need to respect that others may not share my values and ways of seeing things. We all have different values, preferences, and worldviews. There is way too much of people making each other feel bad when they disagree, as in polarizing clashes between political parties. Our world is lacking in humility and respect.

If only we could spend less time trashing each other and more time trying to understand each other.

- *Stand up for yourself.* If someone puts you down for how you think or behave, you can kindly and firmly demand their respect. Sometimes this takes a lot of courage. Be brave. If they continue to disrespect you, disengage. Whatever you do, don't be false. Don't do or say anything that betrays your values or beliefs.

- *Be a light of love.* Stand up to evil and injustice. Speak out. Don't let others engage in racism, gossip, or hate speech without taking a stand. People driven by greed and hate can have a lot of passion. It is important that you be just as passionate in shining a light of love into the darkness of greed, hatred, and ignorance.

- *Seek refuge in a community of like-minded people.* Surround yourself with people who love you for who you are and accept you just as you are.

- *Risk rejection.* Let go of the need for everyone to like you. Don't be afraid to speak your mind. Those who matter won't judge you, and those who judge you don't matter.

Inauthenticity harms you. When you're not true to yourself, you deny yourself. This is painful, for it will leave you with longing. You will then want to numb your longing by addicting.

Authenticity protects your recovery. Make authenticity a way of life. It will take practice and courage, but it is worth it. In the end you will have the satisfaction of living the life you wanted to live, rather than the life someone else wanted you to live. What's more, the world needs you to be you. Being yourself and shining your own light is the best gift you can give to the world.

In Conclusion

You've just learned about the many tools you need to recover from painkiller addiction. Now that you have read this book, it's time to put the principles of healing and recovery into practice. I truly hope that you will work on your recovery every day for the rest of your life. You can stop when you die. If you make just a 1 percent change in your life every month, you will be 100 percent better in six years, and over 1,000 percent better in twenty years!

I suggest you start by getting treatment to get sober, safe, and stable. But don't stop there. Take the principles and practices from this book and build them into your life, one at a time.

Stay motivated. Recovery takes time. You will need to be patient and persistent. You will likely experience plateaus and setbacks. Life is like that. Don't get discouraged. If you keep up your practices, you will continue to slowly grow and heal. You'll notice this better when you look back on your life a year from now and see how much it has improved.

Make it easy for yourself by developing one positive recovery habit at a time. Make them easy to do. For example, once you get a recovery mentor, you might schedule a check-in at a regular time every day to make it easy and predictable. For your spiritual practice, you might start with five minutes a day. For exercise, start with doing five sit-ups and five push-ups. Start small and easy, and build from there.

Set up triggers for your new recovery habits. For example, meditate or pray every morning after you wash your face and brush your teeth. Spend time reading, journaling, and reflecting after your evening meal.

Schedule your life around your recovery. Make your recovery first to make it last. Don't let life get in the way. Watch for complacency. When you think you're all good, you know you're in danger. Remember, you are always wrong to some degree in some ways. That's called "being human." Hopefully, with recovery, you'll gradually become less wrong. May you always be humble in your recovery.

This book is just a start. Set an intention to learn something new every day. Don't stop making an effort to learn and grow. Read, and listen carefully to the wisdom of others.

Are you ready for a miracle? I hope so, because you are about to experience one. Do the work outlined in this book, and you will experience a miraculous transformation of your life. I see it every day, which is why I love this work so much!

You can do this! All it takes is willingness to do the work. Anyone can recover with enough help and support. Ask for help and do the work, and you will be more than fine...you will be fantastic! Won't it be so nice to realize the joyful life that is your birthright! Go for it!

I wish you many blessings on your journey of recovery. May you ride the winds of grace.

With Love,
Michael McGee, M.D.

Affirmations

A ffirmations are positive, realistic statements of you—who you are and who you are becoming. Pick three to five affirmations to recite daily at the beginning of your day during your morning ritual. Repeat them for several weeks until you clearly feel that they are part of who you are. Then pick a new set of affirmations. Use your affirmations to propel your growth.

Affirmations on Self-Worth
- Despite my flaws and failures, I am a sacred being of immeasurable value and worth.
- I accept myself just as I am.
- I love myself.
- I forgive myself.
- I treat myself with compassion when I am hurting.
- I mindfully let go of negative self-judgments.
- I deserve to be happy.
- I am worthy and whole despite feelings to the contrary.

Affirmations on Love and Relationships
- I am loving in everything I say and do.
- Everything I say is loving and kind.
- I don't take what others say and do personally.
- I love for love's sake alone.
- Because I am loving, people find me lovable.
- People's lives are better because of me.

- I unconditionally accept and love everyone exactly as they are.
- I see destructive people as sacred beings who are sick in a destructive way.
- I recognize that if I had another person's genes and life experience, that I would likely act as they act.
- I am loving my family for who they are without expectations.
- I am developing and maintaining a healthy, loving group of friends.
- I am developing and maintaining a vibrant romantic life with my partner.
- I see love everywhere I go.
- My partner and I have a deep mutual understanding.
- I am nonjudgmental.
- I am compassionate.
- I am empathic.
- I am affirming.
- I am hopeful for others.
- I add value to the lives of everyone I encounter.
- I am patient.
- I am forgiving.
- I am generous.
- I am helpful.
- I yield to other's wishes.
- I protect myself from harm.
- I engage only in healthy relationships.
- I am kindly assertive. I stand up for myself.
- I care for my partner, my family, and my friends.
- I take time to connect deeply with others.
- I let others know what I am thinking, feeling, and doing every day.
- I ask for help when I need it.
- I am considerate of other people's needs and feelings.
- I take time to check up on the people I love.
- I build people up.
- I am a channel of love.
- I do what is best for both myself and others.
- I am humble.

- I am respectful.
- Because I radiate confidence and self-respect, others respect me.
- I treat others with reverence, in accordance with their sacredness.
- When I am with others, I look closely and listen carefully.
- I reinforce other people's positive behaviors.
- I allow people to experience the natural painful consequences of their unskillful behavior so that they can learn and grow.
- I am drawing healthy, loving people into my life one day at a time.
- I am honest, trustworthy, and kind.
- I am reliable and helpful.
- I accept others as they are without trying to change them.
- I acknowledge my needs and communicate them clearly to others.
- I deserve to be loved and liked.
- I treat others the way I enjoy being treated.
- My heart is open.
- I am surrounded by people who support me.
- My relationships nurture my recovery.
- My partner is generous and kind.
- I attract only positive people into my life.
- My relationships are grounded in integrity.
- I am safe and well-treated.
- I have the right to be treated with respect.
- I excel at setting boundaries.
- I achieve the perfect balance between self-care and time spent with others.
- I let go of toxic relationships.
- I detach with love.
- I enjoy meeting new people and new people enjoy meeting me.
- I am loved for being exactly who I am.
- I am deserving of love.
- I allow myself to trust in love.
- Love surrounds me, and I give and receive it with ease.

- I release all jealousy and possessiveness.
- I acknowledge my connectedness with all human beings.
- I accept my vulnerability.
- I accept my interdependence.
- I release all resentment, negativity, and remorse.
- I forgive and move forward.
- I am whole.
- I release the need to control people, places, and things.
- I love my job.
- I love my family.
- I love my partner.
- I love my children.
- I love my animals.
- I love myself.
- I love my life.
- I focus on what I have in common with others.
- The more love I give, the more I receive.
- I reclaim my freedom to love.

Affirmations on Work

- I dedicate my work to contributing to others and to making the world a better place.
- I work with gratitude for the opportunity to serve and to make a living.
- I am doing work that I love.
- I am working to find a fulfilling job.
- I further my career with every action I take.
- I am working to create financial abundance.
- I bring value to my coworkers and my boss.
- I bring value to those I serve.
- I strive to do the best at everything I do.
- I do quality work.
- My positive attitude, confidence, and hard work naturally draw in new opportunities.
- I make thoughtful, careful decisions.
- I treat those with whom I work with consideration and respect.
- I do my work with enthusiasm.

- I radiate confidence and success at work.
- I deal with frustrations with a calm, positive attitude.

Affirmations on Well-Being

- I take good care of myself.
- I do nothing to harm myself.
- I cherish and care for myself as if I were my own ideal parent.
- I eat only foods that are good for me.
- I get plenty of rest and sleep.
- I have fun every day.
- I exercise every day.
- I take time to relax.
- I engage in a spiritual practice every day.
- Everything I think, say, and do enhances my health.
- I renounce temporary pleasures that are harmful to me.
- I manage pain with love.

Affirmations on Self-Confidence

- With daily effort, I am achieving all my dreams.
- With practice, I am becoming more and more capable.
- I let go of perfection and practice authenticity.
- I value failures, setbacks, and obstacles as opportunities to learn and grow.
- I face my fears and do what I need to do with courage.
- With positivity, patience, practice, and perseverance, I will achieve my dreams.
- I am just as worthy of success and happiness as anyone else.
- I believe in myself.
- Though I have room to grow, I still like myself.
- I love myself for just who I am, with all my flaws and imperfections.

Affirmations on Finances

- I am learning how to earn, save, and invest money.
- I am frugal.
- I spend money wisely.

- I value money for the security it provides and for the capacity to help others.
- I purchase what I need. I practice contentment, refraining from purchasing everything I want.
- I am working to increase my income by delivering more value to others.

Affirmations on Success

- Every day, I act to realize my key life goals.
- I am 100 percent committed to doing what I need to do to succeed.
- I am dedicated and disciplined.
- I schedule my priorities and follow through on my commitments with discipline.
- I practice my self-improvement rituals daily.
- My actions are in alignment with my life purpose.
- Because of my attitude and efforts, life is getting better every day.
- I am thoughtful, careful, and wise in my actions.
- I take time to reflect on the best course of action.
- I look for the opportunities in difficult situations.
- I am creative.
- I do the next right thing, I act with integrity.
- I am honest, but take care not to use truth as a weapon.
- When I fall, I get back up and persist. I do not give up.
- I am responsible for my life.
- I allow others to help me achieve my goals.
- One way or another, I persist until I accomplish my goals.

Affirmations on Adversity

- I know that pain is temporary, and that difficult times will pass.
- I do not let my trauma define me.
- I recognize that pain is a great teacher, and can transform me into a wiser, more compassionate, and more acceptant person.
- I look to the present moment to help me grow and learn what I need to learn.

- I see that while distress is inevitable, suffering is optional with acceptance.
- I accept all that is outside of my control.
- I see that everything is just as it can only be.
- I see that everything is perfect in its seeming imperfection.
- I am acting to change what I can to improve my situation.
- I am asking for help from others.
- Because of my positive attitude and positive actions, life is getting better every day.
- I am hopeful for both myself and others.
- I am a survivor.
- I choose my attitude and the way I respond to what happens.

Affirmations on Joy, Happiness, and Fulfillment

- I am grateful for all that I have.
- I wake up grateful for the gift of another day.
- This moment is enough, and enough is a feast.
- My life is a blessing and a miracle.
- My life is meaningful.
- I have a purpose.
- Each day, I find reasons to be joyful, to smile and laugh, and to be happy.
- I radiate love, joy, and happiness.
- I practice being mindfully present throughout the day.
- I am at peace.
- I feel connected to all that is.
- I am content.
- I feel connected to a power greater than myself.
- I live a simple life.
- I enjoy learning and growing.
- I enjoy new experiences.
- I experience awe and wonder at the miracle of existence.
- I see the miraculous in the mundane.
- I experience the extraordinary in the ordinary.
- I see that life is sacred.
- I see the sacred in everyone and everything.
- I see beauty everywhere I look.

- I realize that life is about life, and not just about me.
- As I put good out into the world, good comes back to me.
- There is a loving intelligent life force that flows through me.
- My life is filled with grace.

Affirmations for Weight Loss

- I am grateful for my body.
- I am becoming fit and trim.
- I eat only healthful and nourishing foods.
- I eat fewer calories than I burn until I am down to my ideal weight.
- I am physically active.
- I welcome hunger as a sign my body is burning up fat. I smile at my hunger.
- I do not let myself get too hungry.
- I count my calories every day.
- I eat mindfully, stopping just before I am completely full.
- I am excited and hopeful about losing weight.
- I love myself completely, regardless of my weight.
- I enjoy looking good and feeling good.
- I manage my weight to stay healthy and fit.

Affirmations on Authenticity

- Today I will remain true to myself. I will honor my feelings.
- I say what I mean and mean what I say.
- I release the need to wear masks.
- I am loved for being exactly the way I am.
- The more I follow my own heart, the more others love and respect me.
- I let go of the need to please people.
- It is safe to speak my truth.
- I have the right to be inconsistent.
- I have the right to take my time.
- I have the right to take space from others when I need it.
- I have the right to take a different path.
- I am unique in all the world.

- My work reflects my deepest joy.
- My relationships reflect my true values.
- My actions and values are harmoniously aligned.
- I surround myself with people who support my authentic self.
- I honor my inner voice unconditionally.
- I am connected firmly and passionately to my true self.
- I accept myself.
- I allow others to see and know the real me.

Affirmations on Honesty

- My soul heals through honesty and truthfulness.
- I am an honest person.
- I always tell the truth.
- I am known as a truthful, trustworthy individual.
- I find it easy to admit my mistakes.
- I tell the truth even when it is inconvenient.
- I tell the truth even when it is embarrassing.
- I tell the truth even when I fear the repercussions.
- I keep my promises.
- I strive for accuracy.
- I let go of the need to minimize or exaggerate.
- I trust that there are always solutions to my problems.
- I can get my needs met without lying.
- I am emotionally honest.
- I acknowledge my abilities and strengths.
- I live in enduring integrity.
- I do not steal or cheat.
- The more honest I am, the more intimacy I experience with others.
- I face everything and recover.
- When I give my word, it means something.

Affirmations on Growth

- It is safe to shine.
- I realize my potential, and I honor it.
- I allow myself to be in a process.
- I value the journey as much as the destination.

- I release my perfectionism and move forward without fear.
- It's okay to make mistakes.
- I have the courage to follow my dreams.
- I have a bright future.
- I love trying new things.
- I enjoy taking risks and stepping outside of my comfort zone.
- I own all my talents and abilities.
- I embrace the beginner's mind.
- I cultivate new hobbies that I enjoy.
- It is okay to be a late bloomer.
- I am in the right place at the right time doing the right thing.
- I seek out positive role models and mentors.
- I enjoy meeting new people and new people enjoy meeting me.
- Happy, loving people are eager to meet me.
- I reward myself for a job well done.
- I accept praise and appreciation for my work.

Affirmations on Solitude

- I enjoy my own company.
- I am my own best friend.
- I spend some time alone every day.
- I am responsible for my own happiness.
- It is safe to put myself first.
- I enjoy connecting with nature.
- I thrive on my own validation.
- I make time for relaxation, meditation, and adequate sleep.
- I practice healthy boundaries in all my relationships.
- I cultivate an inner sanctuary of peace and serenity.
- I take myself on great dates.
- I am grounded in my senses and in the present moment.
- I enjoy reading and cultivating new hobbies.
- I enjoy getting to know myself better.
- I release the need for drama and chaos in my life.
- I find joy in the simple things in life.
- I use my solitude as another channel for self-discovery.
- I experience solitude as a wonderful adventure.

- I enjoy the silence of my own mind.
- I am comfortable with myself.

Affirmations on Time Management

- I am at peace with time.
- I set boundaries with ease.
- I have plenty of time for each task I need to perform today.
- I love being productive.
- I am in the right place at the right time doing the right thing.
- I find safe harbor in the present moment.
- I allow myself to spend time doing nothing.
- I release the need for chaos around time.
- I release the need to procrastinate.
- I release the need for chronic tardiness.
- I give myself enough time to get where I need to go.
- I create a schedule of balance and harmony.
- Self-care takes the highest priority in my schedule.
- Every day I take time to nurture my creative visions.
- I reward myself for time spent well.
- Beginning today, what serves me stays and what fails me goes.
- Time is a valuable resource that I will spend wisely.
- I am careful to balance work with play and socializing with solitude.
- I have all the time in the world and everything I need.

Affirmations on Self-Care

- Today I will take responsibility for my life, my health, and my happiness.
- I love myself unconditionally.
- I allow myself the proper amount of food, sleep, and enjoyment each day.
- I am worthy.
- I am beautiful.
- I am perfect just as I am.
- I am free from negative substances, people, and energy.
- I find time to exercise every week.
- I nourish my mind and my spirit on a regular basis.

- Each day I do one thing to develop my intellect.
- I take time to discover what is spiritual for me.
- I allow myself to experience and express emotions with ease.
- The more I love myself, the more others love me.
- When I am troubled, I pause to comfort myself and understand my feelings.
- I nourish my body with healthy food every day.
- I enjoy giving to myself as much as others.
- I accept the things I cannot change.
- I am strong physically, mentally, and emotionally.
- Today is my day. There is no person, thing, event, or activity that can destroy this day for me.
- Today is the first day of the rest of my life and I will take notice of the many positive things this day has to offer.

Affirmations on Gratitude

- Every day I appreciate my life more than ever.
- Every day I give thanks for all that blesses my life.
- Mistakes are learning experiences that help me grow.
- With every breath I take, I am bringing more and more gratitude into my life.
- Through the continuous expression of gratitude, I am now living a life of unlimited abundance.
- My grateful heart attracts more of everything I appreciate in life.
- I treat life as the ultimate gift.
- I sincerely appreciate the support I receive from others.
- I take the time to appreciate the simple things in life.
- I thank people often.
- I pay my bills with gratitude.
- I gratefully accept all the good that manifests in my life.
- I am very grateful that I am able to reprogram my life for the better.
- I appreciate all forms of life on this planet.
- I focus on what I have, what I can give, and what I love.
- I honor all that is good about me.
- I own everything about myself.

- I am grateful for my past and use it to uplift others.
- I am grateful for my body, mind, and spirit.
- Through gratitude, I move from surviving to thriving.

Affirmations on Compassion

- I am nonjudgmental and forgiving.
- I forgive myself and others with ease.
- I accept mistakes are part of being human.
- I am kind and gentler toward everyone I meet.
- I see what I can do to contribute.
- I am generous and loving toward myself and others.
- I release the need to bully myself or others.
- I let go of shame and guilt.
- I use positive language and verbal harmlessness.
- I abstain from gossip and character assassination.
- I give and receive compliments with ease.
- I give others the benefit of the doubt.
- Easy does it.
- I am friendly.
- I take an active interest in others.
- I take the time to put a smile on another person's face.
- I do what I can to help those less fortunate than me.
- I let go of grudges and focus on the here and now.
- I let go of the past and live in the present moment.
- I am positive, connected, and I express love with ease.

About the Author

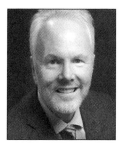

Michael D. McGee, M.D., is the Chief Medical Officer of The Haven, near San Luis Obispo, California; The Haven is a psychiatric treatment facility that specializes in the treatment of addictions. (www.thehaven.com.)

Dr. McGee graduated with distinction from Stanford University with a degree in biology. He received his medical decree from Stanford University School of Medicine and completed his residency in psychiatry at Harvard Medical School, including a chief residency in inpatient psychiatry. He has directed several treatment programs, participated in government-funded outcomes research, and has published in the areas of spirituality, addictions, and clinical treatment.

Dr. McGee is board certified in general psychiatry, addiction psychiatry, and psychosomatic medicine. He has extensive experience in addictions treatment and general adult psychiatry. He is also the author of the multi-award-winning book, *The Joy of Recovery: The New 12-Step Guide to Recovery from Addiction.*

Dr. McGee also has a private practice near San Luis Obispo, where he practices a combination of psychotherapy and psychopharmacology. His approach is eclectic—he draws from a broad spectrum of philosophies. He includes psychospiritual interventions to complement biological, psychodynamic, interpersonal, and cognitive-behavioral interventions. His private practice website is **www.wellmind.com.**

You can learn more about Dr. McGee and his work at **www.drmichaelmcgee.com.**

Consumer Health Titles from Addicus Books

Visit our online catalog at www.AddicusBooks.com

To Order Books:
Visit us online at: www.AddicusBooks.com
Call toll free: (800) 888-4741

For discounts on bulk purchases, call our Special Sales
Department at (402) 330-7493.
Or email us at: info@Addicus Books.com

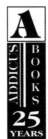

Addicus Books
P. O. Box 45327
Omaha, NE 68145

*Addicus Books is dedicated to publishing consumer health books
that comfort and educate.*